**IF YOU SUFFER FROM
TENSION · ANXIETY · DEPRESSION · INSOMNIA
· OR PAIN, AND SEEK RELIEF THROUGH DRUGS—**

**IF YOU OR ANYONE YOU LOVE HAVE TAKEN
EVEN ONE OF THE DRUGS PICTURED IN THIS BOOK—**

YOU NEED

THE LITTLE BLACK PILL BOOK

Millions of Americans take these powerful drugs to obtain significant medical benefits. Millions more use them for non-medical purposes. Few know that they may become dependent or addicted *even following doctor's orders to the letter*. Or that they may have a genetic predisposition that puts them at extra risk. Or that drug interactions can threaten their life. *Each year, more people die from prescription drugs, obtained legally, than from all illegal substances combined.*

Used properly, *The Little Black Pill Book* could save your life. It synthesizes the most important facts about each drug in a concise, readable entry. Warnings, withdrawal symptoms, and overdose treatment are given special prominence. Also included is information on how drugs work in the body, the psychological side of drug dependence, drugs and the law, dangerous pill lookalikes and drugs of deception, key questions for your doctor—and much more.

**From the producers of the million-copy
bestseller THE PILL BOOK**

The purpose of this book is to provide educational information to the public concerning the majority of psychoactive prescription drugs which are presently utilized by physicians. It is not intended to be complete or exhaustive or in any respect a substitute for personal medical care. *Only a physician may prescribe these drugs and the exact dosage which should be taken.*

While every effort has been made to reproduce products on the cover and insert of this book in an exact fashion, certain variations of size or color may be expected as a result of the photographic process. Furthermore, pictures identified as brand name drugs should not be confused with their generic counterparts, and vice versa. *In any event, the reader should not rely upon the photographic image to identify any pills depicted herein, but should rely solely upon the physician's prescription as dispensed by the pharmacist.*

THE LITTLE BLACK PILL BOOK

BERT STERN	LAWRENCE D. CHILNICK
Producer	Editor-in-Chief

MEDICAL CONSULTANTS

David E. Smith, M.D.	Director/Founder, Haight-Ashbury Free Medical Clinic San Francisco
Richard B. Seymour, M.A.	Director of Training, Haight-Ashbury Free Medical Clinic
John P. Morgan, M.D.	Medical Professor, Director of Pharmacology, School of Bio-Medical Education, CCNY, New York

TEXT BY

Lois B. Morris   Robert Garrett   Ursula Waldmeyer
Lawrence D. Chilnick

PHOTOGRAPHY

Bert Stern
Burt Cohen

PRODUCTION ASSISTANTS

Joy Z. Dermanjian
Ellen Rick

RESEARCH ASSISTANT

Dan Montopoli

BANTAM BOOKS
TORONTO · NEW YORK · LONDON · SYDNEY

QUANTITY PURCHASES

Companies, professional groups, churches, clubs and other organizations may qualify for special terms when ordering 24 or more copies of this title. For information, contact the Direct Response Department, Bantam Books, 666 Fifth Avenue, New York, N.Y. 10103. Phone (212) 765-6500.

THE LITTLE BLACK PILL BOOK
A Bantam Book / December 1983

ISBN 0-553-23786-1

Published simultaneously in the United States and Canada

Bantam Books are published by Bantam Books, Inc. Its trademark, consisting of the words "Bantam Books" and the portrayal of a rooster, is Registered in U.S. Patent and Trademark Office and in other countries. Marca Registrada. Bantam Books, Inc., 666 Fifth Avenue, New York, New York 10103.

PRINTED IN THE UNITED STATES OF AMERICA

O   0 9 8 7 6 5 4 3 2 1

Contents

Tables

Acknowledgments

The staff of *The Little Black Pill Book* wishes to acknowledge the following special people whose time, unselfish help, and dedication has contributed to the value of this book:

Dr. Joanne Baum, Millicent Buxton, Elaine Cohen, Dr. Sidney Cohen, Emma Dermody, Donald K. Fletcher, Dr. George (Skip) Gay, Darryl Inaba, Pharm.D., Dr. Bruce Medd, Stephanie Ross, Dr. Edward Senay, Dr. Donald R. Wesson, and the entire staff of the Haight-Ashbury Free Medical Clinic, whose research efforts and experience were invaluable in the creation of this book.

Rona Fisher Hunter, who successfully fought impossible deadlines to create and produce the insert and cover.

Ned Leavitt and the William Morris Agency, whose expertise and tenacity helped bring an idea to reality.

Jeff Packer and Dave Phillips of Carlyle Chemists, N.Y.C., and William DeNeergaard of the Neergaard Pharmacy, Brooklyn, N.Y., who provided pharmaceutical products for us to photograph.

Toni Burbank and Anne Greenberg, our editors at Bantam, whose perseverance and insights shaped the finished manuscript.

Doreen V. Kagan and Linda Kasak of City College, N.Y.C.

Carol Mackler, who assisted in the assembly of the color insert.

And the following people whose professional skills or editorial assistance have been essential: Janet S. Chilnick, Renée Gelman, Jeff Kabat, James Miglino, Nick Miglino, Maryann Napoli of the Center for Medical Consumer and Health Care Information Inc., Barry Secunda, Barry Sigal, Noel Silverman, Jonathan Skipp, Dr. Irving Slessar, and Dan Strone.

Introduction

by David E. Smith, M.D.
Director/Founder, Haight-Ashbury Free Medical Clinic,
San Francisco, California

Americans take pills at an astonishing rate. More than 2 billion prescriptions a year are filled at a cost of over $10 billion. Twenty percent of these prescriptions are for psychoactive drugs. In addition, a very large number of illicit pills containing psychoactive substances are consumed each year. When these drugs, which often have a profound effect upon the brain, are taken under supervised medical circumstances for appropriate therapeutic purposes they can bring significant benefit to the individual. All too often, however, they are misused when people are misinformed or when they develop addictive disease by continuing to use drugs compulsively despite adverse effects on physical health, mental functioning and economic and social behavior. When misused, pills not only damage the individual but have damaging effects in relation to family, workplace, and other aspects of daily living, including driving. Many thousands of people are unnecessarily injured or killed each year because of the intoxicating effects of psychoactive drugs—particularly when they're combined with alcohol, our country's number one drug problem.

Consumers of drugs that affect the mind are bombarded with a bewildering array of inaccurate or out-of-date information from medical sources, electronic and print media, peers, and so on, so that very often they are totally misinformed.

The Little Black Pill Book provides you with the latest information medical science has about psychoactive drugs, stressing new research on the brain's function and its interaction with drugs. Critical variables of pill abuse are discussed, like the physical characteristics of the individual taking the drug, psychological characteristics, including attitude, and the environment in which the drug is taken. All of these factors can influence the short-term and long-term effects of a drug.

Drug abuse, one of our country's major health problems, is the third leading cause of death, after heart disease and cancer. Our clinical experience over the past 15 years at the Haight-Ashbury Free Clinic has clearly shown that some people can use psychoactive drugs with maximum therapeutic benefit and minimal danger while others, when they begin taking psychoactive drugs, abuse them and damage their physical, mental, and behavioral health. Others repeatedly abuse drugs in a compulsive fashion despite being aware of continued adverse consequences. The pattern of compulsive abuse is seen in approximately 10 million alcoholics in the United States, 2 million nonnarcotic drug abusers, and 1 million narcotic drug abusers.

We now recognize compulsive abuse of psychoactive drugs as an addictive disease. It is apparent from clinical and laboratory research that the disease is a product of genetic factors and environmental influences. A history of drug or alcohol abuse in the family predisposes you to a higher probability of developing addictive disease; you need to be more informed and much more careful before taking pills or other substances that are psychoactive.

When addictive disease develops, treatment is required, which may range from medical management of physical complications to appropriate medical care of an overdose to the administration of other medications to reduce physical dependence.

Getting off is one thing, but staying off is another. For the individual with addictive disease controlled use of psychoactive substances becomes very difficult. Unfortunately, many such consumers deny the negative effects of drugs. Somehow they must be motivated to move into what professionals call recovery, which means living a comfortable and responsible life without the use of psychoactive drugs. To ensure recovery the diagnosis of addictive disease, like that of any other disease, must be based on objective, nonjudgmental criteria. It is important that the individual's need for recovery be balanced with the appropriate use of medicine for a specific, well-documented medical complaint. The information in this book is an invaluable reference for consumers, family, employers, and others whose lives are affected by drug addiction and the problems that accompany rehabilitation.

The Little Black Pill Book provides objective information not only about drugs, but about their complicated interaction with the individual and his environment. We hope you will use this book and your pills wisely, and that if you see you are developing a problem, you will seek help from medical and nonmedical sources.

In an Emergency

A drug overdose; unusual and severe reactions to a pill; symptoms of drug withdrawal. These are life-threatening drug emergencies and require immediate medical attention. Knowing what to do, staying calm, and acting fast can save a life—perhaps your own.

SIGNS OF A DRUG EMERGENCY

The most common signs of drug emergencies are detailed in each drug profile in this book, under the headings "Withdrawal Symptoms" and "Overdose and Treatment." Symptoms can be seemingly mild: a vague sense of discomfort, a headache, feeling tired, or having an upset stomach. With small overdoses of certain pills, such symptoms will probably disappear quickly and cause no further problem. But identical symptoms can also be the beginning of a serious drug emergency that can, in a matter of minutes, result in respiratory collapse, seizures, a heart attack, and coma. It is most unwise for a layperson to assume an adverse reaction is anything less than serious, except when a physician has specifically warned in advance that a reaction is possible, and has given instructions on what to do if it occurs.

Drug emergencies can be very confusing even to a doctor. An amphetamine overdose has symptoms that look like narcotic withdrawal; a barbiturate overdose, on the other hand, can masquerade as stimulant withdrawal. While proper first aid is relatively simple for any drug emergency caused by one of the pills in this book, the appropriate treatment afterward—in an emergency room or doctor's office—can differ greatly depending on the drug involved. Sometimes extensive medical tests are required before a doctor can be sure how much of a drug was taken, or whether someone is experiencing an unusual reaction to a

1

drug. It is therefore essential that a victim of any drug emergency—an overdose, an adverse reaction, or withdrawal—be rushed to a hospital as soon as possible, even while first aid is underway.

Whenever possible, the pill bottle or a sample of the drug involved should accompany the victim to the hospital, so the emergency room staff can quickly identify the medication and begin proper treatment without delay.

GENERAL RULES FOR ALL DRUG EMERGENCIES

1. *Don't delay in phoning for help.* If the area where you live has a special number to call in an emergency, dial it and describe the situation. Or dial "0," (Operator), tell the operator it's an emergency call, and ask to be connected to Poison Control. Or find the number for Poison Control in your phone book, or from Information, and call it directly. When you reach Poison Control, be prepared to tell the person who answers:

• your location;
• what was taken and how much;
• condition of the victim (conscious or sleeping, vomiting, having convulsions, etc.);
• approximate age and weight of the victim;
• chronic medical conditions of the victim (such as diabetes, epilepsy, or high blood pressure), if you know them;
• what medicines, if any, the victim takes regularly.

2. *Never use a second drug.* Don't give a stimulant (even coffee) to a drug overdose victim who seems to be extremely tired, for instance, because the combination can be more dangerous than the original overdose drug.

3. *Assume the worst.* Even if you aren't certain that a person is suffering from an overdose or drug withdrawal, assume he is and get medical help immediately.

4. *Don't be afraid to try to help.* You won't be arrested or otherwise penalized for trying to help during what you believe is a genuine emergency. It's better to apologize later—if you made an honest mistake by rushing someone to the hospital who didn't really have to be treated—than take a chance on letting the person suffer or possibly die. Even if someone doesn't think he needs help, or doesn't want it, call for help anyway, if *you* think it's needed.

5. *Don't try to force an unconscious person to drink or eat.* He could accidentally choke if you do.

IF THE VICTIM IS CONSCIOUS

1. *Ask the victim if an overdose could have occurred,* or whether withdrawal from drugs is the likely cause of the symptoms. If there is any doubt whether overdose or withdrawal is responsible, proceed as though an overdose has occurred. If you are positive that withdrawal is the cause— but *only* if you are positive—then immediately rush the victim to a hospital, following steps 2, 6, and 7 below.

2. *Phone for help immediately.* Call Poison Control, or a hospital or doctor. Tell them, if you know, what drug is involved, and describe the symptoms as well as you can (dizziness, slow or rapid breathing, pinpoint eye pupils, general weakness, etc.). Follow the instructions you receive.

3. *Induce vomiting.* Although in general you should not cause vomiting for poisoning (because some poisons, such as lye, can be more damaging if they are vomited) overdoses of any pill described in this book—and most other medicines—are best treated by forcing the victim to empty his stomach.

Vomiting can be induced by making the victim swallow a spoonful of ipecac syrup (a teaspoon for a child, a tablespoon for an adult) followed by 2 to 3 glasses of water (one glass for a young child). Ipecac syrup is available from most pharmacies in small bottles, and is often included in first-aid kits. If vomiting does not take place within 15 minutes, repeat the dose once.

Vomiting can sometimes be caused by tickling the back of the victim's throat while he is in a "spanking" position (such as a child laying face down over your lap). You should use a spoon or similar household implement; be careful if you use your finger, since you might receive a painful bite if the victim gags.

Not recommended ways to induce vomiting: forcing the victim to swallow mustard powder or large amounts of table salt. Neither method works reliably; excessive salt can make the victim's condition worse.

4. *Administer an antidote.* Activated charcoal is the only safe substance useful as an antidote to overdoses of any pill in this book. When swallowed, it absorbs some of the

drug remaining in the stomach after vomiting. Charcoal is unpleasant to take. It stains the gums and mouth black, feels gritty, and tastes bitter. To make it more palatable, it can be mixed with a small amount of cocoa and swallowed dry, or mixed with water in a dark-colored glass so it doesn't look so bad.

5. *Phone for help again* if it has not arrived.

6. *Talk to the victim* reassuringly, to help keep him conscious and lessen his fears. Give as much emotional support as you can and maintain what is called a "reality base," by identifying yourself over and over so he knows who you are and understands you are trying to help. Maintain eye contact, hug the victim occasionally, and repeatedly tell him he will be all right. Keep him abreast of what's happening around him: "The ambulance will be here any minute"; "The neighbors are waiting outside to bring in the medics."

7. *If help does not arrive* and you have good reason to believe it will not come soon, take the victim to the nearest hospital yourself—by car, taxi, or any other way you can arrange.

IF THE VICTIM IS UNCONSCIOUS OR HAVING CONVULSIONS

1. *Do not try to make the victim vomit.* An unconscious person can choke to death on his own vomit, or on food or liquid he is being forced to ingest.

2. *Find out if the victim is breathing.* Listen closely to the nose, mouth, and chest. If you hear no sound, and see no chest movement, he has probably stopped breathing. The skin turning blue (initially under fingernails and toenails) is another sign that breathing has stopped, or is severely restricted.

3. *If the victim is breathing, phone for help immediately.*

4. *If the victim is not breathing, perform mouth-to-mouth resuscitation.* Mouth-to-mouth resuscitation is easier than you think. Lay the victim on his back. Force the mouth open and check that there are no visible obstructions. Pull the tongue forward if it blocks the throat.

Move the victim's head so the chin juts out, to help open the airway. With one hand, pinch the nose closed. With the other hand firmly holding the chin, keep the mouth open.

Take a deep breath and press your lips to the victim's. Force your air into his lungs as though you're blowing up a balloon. If there is a lot of resistance, and the victim's chest does not expand, check inside the mouth again for obstructions. If you are alone, continue mouth-to-mouth resuscitation for at least 10 minutes before phoning for help, or until the victim starts breathing on his own.

While calling for assistance at the same time you're helping the victim breathe, *do not stop mouth-to-mouth for more than a few seconds at a time*. You can grab the phone, dial "0," then fill the victim's lungs a few more times. Pause again and begin to describe the emergency, then go back to your mouth-to-mouth resuscitation. Complete your explanation between breaths. If a child is the unconscious victim, carry the child close to the phone to minimize time lost in administering mouth-to-mouth.

If possible, have someone else phone for medical help while you continue mouth-to-mouth resuscitation. Do not stop until help arrives, you are too exhausted to continue, or someone else takes over from you.

5. *If convulsions occur* (muscle spasms throughout the body, or suddenly rigid muscles), lay the victim on his stomach, and turn the head to one side to keep him from inhaling anything he might vomit up. Keep him warm with a blanket, and push away from the immediate area anything he might bump into during severe spasms.

6. *Phone for help again* if it has not arrived.

7. *If help does not arrive* and you have good reason to believe it will not come in time, take the victim to the nearest hospital yourself—by car, taxi, or any other way you can arrange. Try to keep an unconscious or convulsive victim lying face down during transport, to lessen the chance of choking.

IF YOU ARE THE VICTIM

1. *Phone for help immediately.*

2. *Unlock your door* if you decide to wait for someone to arrive, so help can reach you without delay if you lose consciousness.

3. *Induce vomiting.* Details of how to make yourself vomit are given on page 3. *Do not* take ipecac syrup if you

think you are close to losing consciousness, since vomiting while unconscious can make you choke.

4. *Take an antidote*. Details of how to use activated charcoal are on pages 3–4.

5. *Phone for help again* if it has not arrived.

6. *Write down the drug name* or keep the pill bottle with you so if you lose consciousness, others will know what drug is involved and can begin treatment without delay.

7. *Do not try to "cure" yourself*, for example by taking a stimulant or drinking coffee to offset a sedative effect. You may do more harm than good.

8. *Do not drive* if you decide not to wait for help. Take a taxi, or try finding someone to drive you to the nearest hospital.

HOW YOU CAN HELP MEDICAL PERSONNEL

1. *Collect information* about the kind of drug involved—whether a barbiturate, amphetamine, tranquilizer, narcotic, or some other drug. This can be vital to a doctor trying to decide on the proper emergency treatment. If possible, find a sample of the drug to bring to the emergency room or give to ambulance attendants. Or try finding an empty pill bottle.

2. *Was the drug legitimate?* Try learning if the drug was purchased from a pharmacy or bought on the street. There are often big differences between legitimate drugs and street drugs, and the source can be important to a doctor's decision on how to treat the victim.

3. *What was taken with the drug?* If you can discover whether the drug was used with alcohol, cocaine, marijuana, another drug, or any other substance, tell the medical personnel.

4. *How much was taken?* Try to determine how much of the drug was used, and how recently.

5. *The victim's drug history* can be extremely important to a doctor deciding how tolerant the victim is to the drug involved in the emergency. If you know how long the victim has been using a specific drug, and the amounts, such information may save his life.

BE PREPARED

Every household should be ready for a drug emergency. Now is the proper time—*before* an emergency arises—to do the following:

1. Get the phone number of your local Poison Control center and write it down near your telephone with other emergency phone numbers such as fire and police.

2. Find out NOW which hospital is closest to you, and think about how you can get there quickly in an emergency.

3. Buy a 1-ounce bottle of ipecac syrup at your pharmacy, and make sure you understand how to use it properly. Ask the pharmacist. Keep it where you can find it quickly in an emergency.

4. Learn how to give mouth-to-mouth resuscitation. Practice at least once with a friend so you are not so nervous in an emergency.

5. Keep all medicines out of the reach of children, who are the most frequent victims of accidental pill overdoses. Put drugs in a locked cabinet if possible.

6. Never remove the labels from pill containers. They can provide vital information in case of an emergency.

7. Discard all medicines after you no longer need them.

8. Never take a pill—or any medication—without knowing what it is, and what its possible effects on you may be.

How to Use This Book

If you suffer from tension or anxiety and depression and seek relief through drugs, you need *The Little Black Pill Book*.

If you face fatigue or insomnia and use pills for treatment, you need this book.

If you are plagued by pain and want up-to-the-minute information about the most potent pain killers available, you need this book.

Used properly, *The Little Black Pill Book* can save your life. It can keep you from getting hooked on a drug prescribed, in good faith, by your doctor. Or it can prevent you from becoming dangerously involved with pills you decide to take on your own.

Most of the several hundred drugs described in this book are psychoactive, which means they affect your central nervous system. Psychoactive drugs include most stimulants, tranquilizers, and narcotic analgesics (pain killers), as well as a few other broad categories of drugs. All are powerful medications that can drastically change your perception of reality. They are used legitimately, of course, to treat recognized medical ailments. But they are also used for a multitude of nonmedical purposes, such as improving sexual performance or providing a "high."

The Little Black Pill Book is intended as a guide to the medical uses of pills. But we recognize that drug abuse is widespread, and this book also gives you the straight story about pills commonly used for "recreational" or other nonmedical purposes.

The Little Black Pill Book is divided into three main sections:

I. Important chapters about the many aspects and dangers of drug use and abuse in the 1980s, whether caused by a doctor's improper prescription, by your own decision to use a drug, or by your individual response to a drug.

II. Easy-to-read profiles of the most abused pills in the country.

III. An extensive color index of pills, using actual-sized, color-coded pictures which can help you identify drugs by sight—including a section of lookalike, or counterfeit pills. This section will refer you to detailed information elsewhere in the book about the pill you've identified.

SECTION I: PILL ABUSE IN THE 1980s

This section will help you understand how pills are being used—and abused—in this decade. You will learn whether your genetic makeup, or your family history, makes you a likely candidate for addiction. And you will learn what addiction really means.

Whenever you take a pill, it has certain effects in your body. Sometimes you will feel nothing while the chemicals in the pill spread throughout your body until they are broken down into components that your system can eliminate. Other pills, including the psychoactive medicines described in this book, have a more distinct impact on your senses: while they are in your system you may feel elated, perhaps, or tired, or confused. This section will explain how pills work inside your body, and tell you how physical addiction takes place.

The influence your surroundings may have on your addiction potential—your neighborhood, your friends, your attitude toward pills—is also detailed in this section. The pressures put on you by people you work with or spend time with in the evening can lead to addiction as surely as your physical reaction to a drug. This section will explain the why, and the how, with the help of case histories of people who have abused pills.

Some of the case histories are based on clearly established patterns of drug use, but do not refer to specific people. Others describe the experiences of real people; here, names and other identifying details have been changed.

These case histories demonstrate that drug abuse is not just a matter of taking too many pills. It involves individuals, using particular drugs at particular times and under specific circumstances, perhaps mixing drugs unwisely, or perhaps even *not* using them when they are needed. Each person's history of drug use, or abuse, is different in detail, but the case histories will help you understand broad similarities and overall trends in the use of pills.

Specifically, this section will tell you:

• what drug abuse really means and how it occurs. Did you know that some people, after taking only a few pills, become physically or psychologically dependent on them? Others require several times the dosage—and weeks or months more of usage—before dependence begins. Which group do you belong to? This section will help you find the answer;

• what is meant by "abuse," "tolerance," "cross-addiction," and other words frequently misused even by drug specialists;

• what kinds of drugs cause physical dependency and/or addiction; and which ones result in psychological dependency;

• how you can avoid addiction *without* giving up pills;

• how to cope with a drug problem if it has already occurred in your family;

• what laws affect your pill use, and some commonly asked questions and answers about pills and the law;

• what a doctor is obliged to tell you about the pills he prescribes;

• what information about pills you should be getting from your pharmacist.

SECTION II: DRUG PROFILES

Easy-to-read profiles of the most abused prescription drugs in the United States comprise this section. The drug profiles have been grouped according to their main similarities:

Stimulants. Often called "speed," these can keep you awake for long periods of time and cause some degree of euphoria. Most are amphetamine compounds, first used decades ago to clear stuffy noses and sometimes prescribed today to help people lose weight.

Sedatives. These include sleeping pills and tranquilizers, among them many of the most widely abused medications ever manufactured. Barbiturates, sometimes employed in suicide attempts, are described, along with drugs that act like barbiturates but are chemically different. Other sedatives in this section are benzodiazepines—like Librium and

Valium—which are safer than barbiturates but still very dangerous if misused.

Narcotic Analgesics. These powerful drugs are exceptionally effective in relieving pain, but are also dramatically addictive—even deadly—when used improperly. They include codeine, morphine, and opium.

Antipsychotics. These drugs are more often abused by physicians who prescribe them improperly than by individuals taking them without medical advice. Although they are extremely valuable in treating some forms of mental illness, some of these drugs are used to subdue psychiatric patients for the convenience of a hospital's staff, rather than to benefit the patient. Their side effects can be extremely unpleasant and dangerous and often cannot be reversed when the drugs are discontinued.

Antidepressants. Used to treat severe depression, the tricyclic antidepressants are among the most potent drugs in use today, and can cause many dangerous side effects. Serious illness, even death, can result from using them without full medical supervision.

Each group of drugs is introduced by such general information as their history (when they were first created, and why) or their most serious dangers. Some groups are further divided according to chemical similarities. Thus the chapter on sedatives has a general introduction, then more detailed introductions to the five categories of sedatives: barbiturates, barbiturate combinations, barbituratelike sedatives, benzodiazepines, and benzodiazepinelike sedatives. The chapter on antipsychotic drugs has only one introduction because all the drugs in the group are chemically similar. The groupings reflect not only chemical similarities but also similarities of usage, side effects, and interactions with other drugs.

Following the introductions come further details about the various drug families, keyed to these main features:

1. *Precautions*: Any drug can harm you if you are unusually sensitive to it. Here you will be alerted to possible allergic reactions and other important precautions you should be aware of when taking any drug in the group. The precautions are serious warnings you should *always* heed, such as warnings against driving a car if a drug can slow your reactions to an emergency on the road.

2. *Interactions*: Some drugs should never be taken if you are already taking certain other drugs. Drugs can also react adversely with alcohol, certain foods, and even sunlight. Such warnings will be found here, and are also summarized in a table on pages 97–99.

3. *Common side effects*: These are the side effects that should be expected when using the drug. Common side effects may vary in duration and intensity depending on drug dosage and setting. They may also vary depending on what other drugs, food, or other substances you have used along with the drug. You will not find a complete list of every reported side effect: with some drugs, the list could be several pages long. We have selected only the most frequently experienced side effects for inclusion. If you experience a side effect not listed contact your physician immediately.

4. *Serious adverse effects*: These are more unusual—and more serious—side effects of a pill that should cause you concern. If you experience any of these effects, *call your doctor immediately*.

5. *Dependence and addiction*: This very important part of the drug profile alerts you to dependence potential, or chance for addiction. Some drugs can rapidly cause physical dependence; if you abruptly stop using them, you may experience serious withdrawal symptoms such as hallucinations or even coma. Others seldom result in physical dependence but can lead to serious psychological dependence; you may crave the drug even though you are not suffering from withdrawal pains.

6. *Withdrawal symptoms and treatment*: No one should treat drug withdrawal without the help of a trained medical professional. Here you will learn how to recognize withdrawal symptoms when they occur, and the most commonly used treatments—which can vary from those only possible in a hospital's intensive care room to simple verbal support until the symptoms fade.

7. *Overdose symptoms and treatment*: The most commonly observed symptoms of drug overdose are described, together with immediate steps you, and a physician, must take during an overdose emergency. If you suspect an overdose, *the victim must be rushed immediately to a hospital for treatment. Bring the pill bottle if possible, so that the emergency room staff can quickly identify the drug*

involved and begin proper treatment without delay. Every overdose is a medical emergency. If you suspect an overdose, don't delay. If you are mistaken, you can apologize later; if an overdose has really occurred, you can save a life.

8. *Usage in pregnancy*: Many drugs cross the placenta of a pregnant woman and enter the unborn infant's blood system. Some can have a serious effect on the fetus; a few may cause birth deformities and brain disorders in the newborn. Because there is almost always a gap of several days to a few weeks between the time of conception and confirmation of pregnancy, women who think they may be pregnant—or who are hoping to become pregnant—should avoid any drug that has the slightest chance of adversely affecting a fetus.

9. *Usage during breast feeding*: Just as some drugs can pass from a pregnant woman to her unborn baby, many drugs can be transferred from a nursing mother to her young child during breast feeding.

10. *Usage by the elderly*: People in their 60s and beyond usually metabolize food more slowly than younger men and women; they also metabolize drugs more slowly. Since drugs take longer to be eliminated from their systems, the elderly face an increased probability that the drugs they take can reach potentially dangerous levels.

11. *Usage by children*: Children are usually more sensitive than adults to the drugs described in this book. Recommended dosages are often lower, and children must be watched for side effects which they may not even realize are occurring.

Individual Drug Listings

Following the general description of the drug family come individual listings of each drug:

1. *Generic and brand names*: Most of the drugs in *The Little Black Pill Book* are listed first under their generic, or chemical, names, and then by one or more brand names. Drug manufacturers usually market pills under a brand name, which may have a syllable (or a few letters) that sounds like the chemical name. For example, *dex*troamphetamine sulfate is the generic name for a stimulant called *Dex*ampex by one manufacturer; chlordia*ze*poxide hydro-

chloride is the generic name for a popular tranquilizer called *Ze*tran by one maker; chl*or*promaz*ine* hydrochloride is the chemical name for an antipsychotic drug one manufacturer calls Th*ora*zine.

Some drugs, however, are listed by brand name first, followed by the chemical names of their ingredients. (This is the case with barbiturate combination products, where several drugs are joined to make a single brand-name pill. Butseco, for example, is the brand name of one drug made up of phenobarbital, butabarbital sodium, and secobarbital sodium). Brand-name listings avoid the confusion which would be inevitable if combination drugs were listed several times, under the chemical name of each ingredient.

The brand names are followed by the short form of the name of the manufacturer. Companies' complete names and addresses are listed in the current Physicians' Desk Reference (PDR) or similar publications available at your library or through your druggist or doctor.

After the name or names in the drug profiles, you will find an indication of the drug's classification by the federal government according to its potential for abuse. A few drugs in this book carry no such designations since the government does not consider them addictive; but they require prescriptions. Drug classifications appear as Schedule I through V (see chapter 7).

2. *Street names*: If a pill has a common street name, it will appear here.

3. *Most commonly prescribed for*: These are the approved medical indications for each drug. Most drugs are prescribed for certain symptoms, but often a drug may be used in combinations for quite different reasons. Check with your doctor if you are not sure why you were given a certain pill.

4. *General information*: Any important information that makes this particular drug different from other chemically related drugs.

5. *Onset and duration*: Where appropriate, the profile tells you how quickly the pill takes effect, and how long its effect lasts.

6. *Dosage*: We list the maximum and minimum amounts of a drug usually prescribed; however, you may be given substantially different dosage instructions by your doctor. It is important to check with a physician if you are at all

confused about how often to take a pill, when to take it, or why a dosage was prescribed that is different from those mentioned in this book. Do not change the prescribed dosages on your own; call your doctor first. Dosages differ for various age groups, and for different usages of a particular drug; information about this is provided here.

7. *Available sizes*: Sizes of tablets and capsules are listed at the end of each profile. Some pills release their contents slowly into your system; they are called "sustained-release" pills.

Important note: If you are using this book to look up information about a particular drug, we urge you to read *all* the information about that drug. Do not simply check the portion of the drug profile that gives you the brand names, the reasons the pill is most often prescribed, and the usual dosages. Read also the introductory material pertaining to all the drugs within the same chemical class. If you read only individual drug profiles, you may miss a key warning about the pill, and suffer seriously because of it.

SECTION III: COLOR INDEX

This section is designed to help you identify pills by their color, shape, and size.

While every effort has been made to depict the drugs accurately, certain variations of size or color may occur as a result of the photographic process. Also, you should never rely solely upon the photographic image to identify any pill, but should check with your pharmacist if you have any questions about identification.

Some people may view a peach-colored pill as pink; others will see it as orange. If you don't see the pill you're looking for in one section, check the other sections where colors are similar.

Although many dosage sizes and shapes are included, not all dosage forms of a specific drug can be shown—only the most popular.

Most although not all of the drugs in the color index can be matched with the pill you are trying to identify by comparing the following:

• the imprinted company logo (e.g., "Lilly," "Roche");

- the product strength (e.g., "250 mg.," "10 mg."), which is often printed on pills;
- the product code number (if imprinted).

Because many generic pills look the same as their brand-name counterparts, some manufacturers have started printing the product name on the tablets and capsules.

The color index also contains a section on lookalike drugs, which will help you identify them. Lookalike drugs are either fake prescription drugs or legal over-the-counter products made to look like the real thing (see chapter 8).

THE BEST WAY TO USE THIS BOOK

Look up the drug you are concerned about, either by checking the index or turning to the chapter that deals with similar drugs.

Read about the *whole* class of drugs that includes the one you're most interested in.

Check the individual drug profiles to understand how drugs that are closely related still have important differences.

Read section I to understand fully your own risk of drug dependence or addiction, and to get guidelines on safe drug use.

If you have any further questions about your pills, or if something you read in *The Little Black Pill Book* does not jibe with instructions you have been given, contact your doctor or pharmacist. Make it a rule to know everything you can about what you're taking—before you take it.

I
Pill Abuse in the 1980s

1
What Is Drug Abuse—and Who's at Risk?

Each year more people die from prescription drugs, obtained legally, than from all illegal substances combined.

Tranquilizers, muscle relaxants, sleeping pills, stimulants, appetite suppressants, pain killers, antipsychotics, and antidepressants—most of them obtained legitimately to ease the agonies of life—account for more emergency room visits and deaths than heroin, cocaine, PCP, marijuana, speed, and LSD. According to a report to Congress by the General Accounting Office (GAO) in October 1982, "The abuse of prescription drugs, most of which are obtained at the retail level, results in more injuries and deaths than all illegal drugs combined."

Not all drug misuse or abuse lands somebody on an emergency room trolley or a coroner's slab. But drug treatment programs and detoxification units are finding themselves with a new kind of client on their hands: the average, middle-class, employed, mainstream you-or-me with a pill problem. Most of these pills are by prescription from doctors or dentists. The abusers get hooked on them despite the best of intentions—and despite symptoms and warning signs of drug abuse that they don't recognize and respond to early enough. They don't think the drugs they take are capable of being abused, or themselves capable of abusing them.

THE TRADITIONAL vs. THE NEW ABUSER

Traditionally (and as used in the GAO report), drug abuse is defined as any "nonmedical use" of a substance (usually a psychoactive drug, one which affects the central nervous

19

system) for "psychic effect," dependency, or suicide. Anybody who takes a pill in a way that differs from a doctor's expressed orders is by this definition an abuser: for example, the ad executive who bums a tranquilizer from a colleague before pitching a new multimillion-dollar client; the college student who takes a pill to improve sex; or the comedian who keeps taking his pain medication long after his pain is gone, first because it makes getting up on stage or in front of a camera that much easier, and then because if he doesn't take it he doesn't feel normal. Jerry Lewis, who reveals this side of his past in his autobiography, is just one of a number of celebrities going public in recent years with a pill or mixed-substance abuse problem (or getting publicly busted for illegal possession).

Of course, entertainers have long been media favorites for their "recreational" drug taking: not the least are late-greats like Judy Garland, Janis Joplin, Elvis Presley, and John Belushi. And professional sports stars are lately vying with Hollywood for who gets the biggest cocaine use headlines. Less expected (although as widely reported) was the confession by former first lady Betty Ford that she too had a drug problem. Hers was a grievously common pattern: pain killers and tranquilizers prescribed on a constant basis for fourteen years, to prevent the spasms and pain of a pinched nerve in her neck and arthritis, all combined with alcohol. Though perhaps some people viewed her inability to stop taking the drugs as "weak," in fact once her drug-taking pattern was established, her body required these chemicals to maintain a physiological equilibrium. Any attempt to quit would have thrown her into severe and perhaps life-threatening withdrawal—worse, with the combination of drugs she was taking, than from heroin. In other words, Betty Ford was hooked. In order to quit, she required medical detoxification procedures and close supervision at the Long Beach Naval Hospital's Drug and Alcohol Rehabilitation Center.

Betty Ford did not set out to abuse drugs. Hers was "nonmedical use," however, in that she combined her drug taking with alcohol.

Georgette Bowen (not her real name) is no celebrity. Her story would never make headlines, yet it is startling, for Georgette followed her doctor's orders to the letter. He prescribed Ativan, a drug in the same chemical class as

Valium, for symptoms of anxiety and sleeplessness, possibly associated with menopause. Georgette was fifty at the time. Her doctor warned her not to mix Ativan and alcohol, which wasn't a problem because after her childhood experiences with her alcoholic father, she hardly ever drank; she was rather strongly against recreational drugs of any kind. She wasn't even sure that she wanted to take tranquilizers, but her doctor assured her that 3 milligrams a day was a reasonably modest dose. And the Ativan did help her sleep, which after a long siege of insomnia was a great relief.

Georgette took her pills, though never as regularly as the doctor ordered. After less than a year she decided suddenly to discontinue them. Five days later, Georgette's insomnia returned with a vengeance. Even worse, periodically during the day her whole body would begin to shake. She could hardly eat. She remembered all too well her father's alcoholic DTs. Georgette thought she must be going crazy. Her husband, a policeman, wondered about that himself. Georgette called her doctor and he advised her to return to the Ativan. Sure enough, her symptoms disappeared. Two weeks later she tried to stop again, but the terrible symptoms—worse than what she had suffered before she began the original course of Ativan—resumed. Again the doctor told her to go back on the pills. When her husband questioned whether the symptoms could have anything to do with the drug itself, the doctor said no, not at that low a dose. The doctors at the emergency drug clinic where Georgette ended up disagreed; they said that Georgette was in withdrawal.

THE "TEN-PERCENTERS"

Georgette, with her family history of alcoholism, is one of the 10 percent of the population addiction research has recently shown to have a "psychobiological predisposition" to drug dependency and addiction at *normally prescribed dosages*.

Anybody can develop a physical or psychological dependency on a psychoactive drug after taking high doses of it over a long enough period of time. And anybody can become addicted to a drug who uses it compulsively whatever the terrible consequences. But people like Georgette can get hooked and become addicts without doing anything to "deserve" it. They can get hooked despite following doctor's orders exactly. They can get hooked *because* they follow doctor's orders exactly.

With a parent who had a history of substance abuse, Georgette was 35 times as much at risk of dependency and addiction as the rest of the population. If both of her parents had had drug or drinking problems, Georgette would have been 400 times as much at risk. Georgette's family history predisposed her to addiction to a prescription drug that may have been safe for a person with a different genetic makeup. Because her doctor was uninformed about these important facts, Georgette became a "new addict."

Lack of information, misinformation, inconsistent and contradictory attitudes toward prescription vs. recreational drug taking—all have created an environment in which anyone who takes a pill today for pain or mood or tension or sleeplessness is potentially at risk. If Georgette, with her strict scruples about drug taking, could slip blindly into drug abuse, "so could the Easter Bunny," commented her 25-year-old, marijuana-smoking son.

HOW WE GOT HERE—A SHORT HISTORY OF DRUG USE

Since the beginnings of human history, we (as the American Medical Association's *Drug Abuse, A Guide For the Primary Care Physician*, by Bonnie Baird Wilford, puts it) "have used an almost endless variety of spirits, herbs and potions to relieve ... feelings of sadness, loneliness, tension and boredom." Not to mention our pain and sleeplessness, or our desire for spiritual oneness with the universe.

Many of the substances whose use has been severely restricted or declared illegal in this century have been around—growing on bushes and trees or popping up out of the ground—forever. Alcohol flows freely throughout the Bible; Noah, for one, rather overdid it. The Greeks raised wine to the level of godliness in the form of Bacchus. And in the *Odyssey*, created sometime before 700 B.C., Homer described an experience that might have come from a shot of Demerol (and probably came from some naturally occurring opiate, such as the poppy, from which Demerol is derived and which still grows in abundance in that part of the world): "Now Helen, daughter of Zeus, turned her thoughts elsewhere. Straightaway, she cast into the wine of which they drank, a drug which quenches pain and strife and brings forgetfulness to every ill."

Coca leaves (source of cocaine) have been the elixir of choice in South America since prehistoric times. Opium has been used in Mediterranean countries for thousands of years; it made its way to China in the 1800s. These drugs and others came into Western cultures as the world began to be explored. Europeans discovered caffeine in coffee, nicotine in tobacco, opiates, cocaine—Sigmund Freud, in his early days as a neurologist, was moved to ecstasy (personally and professionally) over cocaine's properties. Marijuana was rapidly accepted for medical purposes in 19th-century England after a British doctor in India reported its usefulness for migraine headaches, arthritis, and menstrual cramps. American doctors began to import it from the Near East as a pain killer, for which it was soon routinely dispensed. Opium and its derivatives (such as morphine, heroin, and codeine) also made their way here, often appearing in patent medicines such as "snake oil." Such products caused widespread dependency and addiction; in 1914 Congress passed the Harrison Narcotic Act to restrict the availability of opiates and cocaine to medical practitioners. Physicians who attempted to help addicts by providing maintenance doses were arrested. By 1919 no narcotics were available legitimately in the U.S. A different type of addict—the criminal—was created as addicts turned to illegal sources.

But then as now, American society, founded on the hard-work ethic, demonstrated strongly mixed feelings about recreational drug use. Even alcohol came under the gun during Prohibition, only to be resurrected after its ban caused gang wars, multimillion-dollar bootleg operations, and little compliance.

Officially in the U.S. we condemn individuals or groups who defy dominant drug norms, labeling them "sinners, criminals, social deviants or emotional cripples" (*Drug Abuse, A Guide for the Primary Care Physician*). Marijuana had been used principally by southern blacks, Mexican laborers, and whites with cultural interests such as jazz that brought them in contact with users. In 1925 its use was made a felony in Louisiana; other states quickly followed. The Marijuana Tax Act of 1937 established federal control over the drug, and in 1951 the Boggs Amendment made penalties for sale or possession of marijuana equivalent to those for narcotics infractions. Until recently even medical use of marijuana was forbidden.

This view toward casual use of drugs and casual users persists—despite the widespread change in attitude toward mind-altering drugs that took place first among the young and spread like a prairie fire throughout the remaining population in the 1960s. (National Institute on Drug Abuse statistics reveal that by 1979 marijuana was third in frequency of use behind alcohol and cigarettes.) In 1950 illicit drug use was confined to heroin and there were some 100,000 users, according to AMA estimates, principally in ghettos. In 1980 there were "tens of millions," says Bonnie Baird Wilford in the AMA guide, from all areas of society and levels of income, all ages, and taking all available drugs. Including prescriptions.

Unlike our attitude toward "recreational use," there is nothing equivocal about America's attitude toward prescription drugs: we welcome them with open arms and open mouths. Drugs are the mainstay of modern medicine, psychiatry included; never before have doctors been able to deal so effectively with what hurts us most and disturbs our functioning. In the realm of pain there is now a drug, Fentanyl, which is 50 to 100 times as effective as morphine. (It has other uses typifying the modern drug dilemma: the late Barney Clark, recipient of the first permanent artificial heart, was anesthetized with it prior to his surgery; under the name of China white it is sold like heroin on the street.) There are whole new classes of drugs which can influence psychosis and soothe the anxiety and depression which mark the worst of its suffering.

Anxiety and depression are, of course, like physical pain, inseparable from being alive and human. Anything which can soften their blow, encourage serenity, provide balance in a world which seems entirely to lack it, we swallow with relief.

America prefers to get its mind drugs from the pharmacy rather than the drug pusher. There are *20,000* potentially abusable psychoactive drug products that fall under federal control (federal drug schedules are explained in chapter 7). More than *20 billion* doses of them are distributed through legitimate channels each year. This does not include substances that are illegally manufactured and sold on the street, estimated at another several million doses. In 1981 Americans spent $40–$50 per capita on these legal "head drugs."

WHAT IS DRUG ABUSE?

Thus most of America takes drugs—and the confused attitudes about what drug taking is have fostered the climate in which the actual dimensions of the drug-abuse problem have not been recognized. Sadly, a lot of unsuspecting folks who would never dream of "doing drugs," like Georgette Bowen, find themselves wrestling with a drug problem.

Lack of information is perhaps the greatest contributor to drug abuse. Downright myths (ten of which are listed on pages 29–33) shape public and personal behavior. The following chapters reveal the facts of drug use and abuse. The 1960s spawned both a new wave of drug taking and a new generation of scientists to study it. In the ensuing decades they have built a body of knowledge, grounded solidly in theory and experience, out of which it is possible at last to separate the facts from the persistent inaccuracies.

The principal prevailing misconception is that it's the drug you take—not how much you take, under what conditions, or with what other substances—that accounts for drug abuse. In fact all psychoactive substances, from a shot of heroin to that mild sleeping pill your doctor kindly prescribed for you, are capable of producing abuse. And in every case abuse can be avoided—you can have your pills and take them too. But you (and the drug prescribers) must be aware of all the risk factors and which among them are under your control, which not. How all these facts and factors figure into the complex process of drug abuse is detailed in the next two chapters and pill by pill in section II of *The Little Black Pill Book*. First, however, they must be seen in the context of what drug abuse really is.

THE MANY DEFINITIONS OF DRUG ABUSE

The traditional definition of drug abuse given above—nonmedical use—may do more harm than good. Practical and repeated experience tells Marvin the accountant that taking a Quaalude to mellow out at the end of a grueling tax season is not likely to hurt him. He loses respect for the powers-that-be who tell him he's doing something awful to himself, pays no attention to antidrug messages, and is lured into a false confidence about the "safety" of the drug. Likewise, Georgette Bowen, who is following doctor's orders, has no way of appropriately evaluating or coping with the harm she has come to.

What about some other common definitions of drug abuse? Is drug abuse—

- use of an illegal drug as opposed to a legal one?
- use of any substance to the point of intoxication?
- use of any drug to the point of intoxication that's obnoxious?
- use of a substance in a way or for a reason of which society as a whole does not approve?
- use to the point of addiction?

Most of these definitions are socially, culturally, or legally determined. They have neither stemmed the tide of drug abuse nor helped anyone deal with its realities. Neither have definitions which focus solely on the amount of drug taken. "At the one extreme," states the AMA guide, "excessive intake of any substance is termed drug abuse. Under this rubric would fall the 10-cup-a-day coffee drinker, the two-pack-a-day cigarette smoker, and the four-in-one-gulp aspirin taker. At the other extreme, only chronic ingestion that leads to a state of physical and psychological dependence is termed drug abuse. This definition rejects intermittent use, which accounts for perhaps 75% of all psychoactive drug taking."

THE DEFINITION THAT MAKES MOST SENSE

Here is a more common-sense definition of drug abuse, which is now being used by some addiction researchers and specialists providing assistance to people with drug problems. The advantage of this definition is that you can use it to identify and bring your own drug use behavior under control.

Drug abuse is a single episode or repeated pattern of substance use to the point where it seriously interferes with your health, or your economic or social functioning.

The *consequences* of your drug use, in other words, are what make it abuse.

USE, MISUSE, AND ABUSE

Carl Henderson and his wife, Sally, live in a southern California town. Carl's doctor recently prescribed a benzodiazepine tranquilizer to be used in conjunction with blood pressure therapy. He took his Serax four times a day like a good patient. On the fourth day Carl had a fight with his wife before leaving for work. The more he thought about it during the day, the more upset he got. So before getting in his car to go home, he took another two pills just to calm down. At this point Carl is guilty of drug *misuse*: his doctor had not prescribed the pills for Carl to take at will. As he drove out of the parking lot, he barely realized just how groggy he was. By the time he did it was too late; the car in front of him on the freeway had put on its brakes and Carl cracked right into it. He broke his nose and almost lost an eye. *Abuse?* Yes, because the consequences to Carl's health were serious. That experience was enough to convince Carl not to meddle with the dosage—or if he did, not to drive.

Carl's wife, Sally, however—and this was one of the reasons for their battle that morning—was taking pills to get high. *Drug misuse.* Valium and Miltown (she was getting them from two doctors) plus a couple of drinks—apparently she'd been doing it for months while he was away at work. He began to notice that she was letting the housework and shopping go, letting herself go, always half-asleep, and deeply depressed in the mornings. *Drug abuse.* A few days before his car accident Carl had come home early and found her flat out on the couch with an empty gin bottle, the two containers of pills, and their seven-month-old screaming in a messy diaper in his crib. He demanded that Sally stop. She said she would but she didn't; in fact she got hold of some cocaine, which Carl didn't know about. The morning of his accident he had hollered at her, "I knew you'd turn out this way, a pillhead, a drunk—you're just like your parents." Exactly. Sally Henderson's family history had helped her join the ranks of the "new addict." She couldn't stop taking the drugs: she had become a compulsive drug user.

Meanwhile, the Hendersons' neighbor Harvey was going crazy from their fighting—he was having a hard enough time trying to work without all that racket. Harvey was a screenwriter. He worked at home. He had been stuck for about a month and a half on a script that was really important to his career. He was able to write, but he felt it just wasn't going right. He'd taken amphetamines when he was in college to get his thesis done. His wife mentioned that she still had about forty Dexedrines left from a prescription a diet doctor had given her years before. Harvey took one and was hot at the typewriter within two hours. *Misuse.* He took one, sometimes two a day and quickly ran out. His wife, Joan, called the doctor and asked for a refill, but he said sorry, he didn't prescribe them anymore. Now Harvey was in a panic—but he couldn't get himself to replenish his supply from the street, or to buy cocaine, for that matter, though a colleague offered to sell him some. Try marijuana, someone else suggested, but Harvey had a thing against that drug too. He sat down and tried to tough it out at the typewriter. To no avail. Now Harvey not only couldn't write badly—he couldn't write at all. *Abuse.*

Drug misuse, abuse, and addiction are not simple events. We are affected by the drugs, by our bodies, by our genetic makeup, and by a series of personal and environmental variables that differ for everyone. These factors contributed as much to the Hendersons' personal problems and to Harvey's writer's block as to their resulting abuse of drugs in order to cope with them. To understand, avoid, and ultimately deal with drug abuse, you must begin to assess your own constellation of variables.

TEN MYTHS OF DRUG ABUSE

1. **MYTH: Most of those who become hooked on drugs have an underlying addictive personality.**

   REALITY: Research has shown that there is no greater incidence of psychological problems among addicts than there is among those who take drugs with less consequence. If anything, there is an addictive *physiology*. Although emotional problems may contribute to why a person seeks or is given drugs, the mechanism of dependency and addiction is predominantly biochemical, resulting from many predictable factors.

---

2. **MYTH: Addiction occurs principally among people with weakened, rebellious, or otherwise negative social values. Therefore, most addicts come from ghetto and/or criminal populations.**

   REALITY: Attitudes, values, and treatment by society (as detailed in chapter 3) contribute to setting the stage for drug abuse and addiction. But so do your genes. Research conducted over the last ten years reveals that 10 percent of the entire population—from the ghetto to the country club—is psychobiologically predisposed to drug dependency and addiction. This finding begins to explain why one person will get hooked on a drug and another not, at the same dose. For this 10 percent, drugs are potentially more habit-forming than they are for the rest of the population.

   If you have a family history of alcoholism or drug abuse, you are within this 10 percent segment. If one parent has or ever had a substance problem, even if it was successfully coped with before you were conceived, you are 35 times as likely to develop a dependency and addiction problem with alcohol or drugs once you are exposed to them. If both parents have that history, you are 400 times as likely.

---

3. **MYTH: The drugs that are the most habit-forming and cause the worst withdrawal problems are the "street" drugs like heroin, cocaine, marijuana, and PCP.**

   REALITY: All psychoactive substances, prescription pills included, are capable of producing dependency and withdrawal (defined in detail in chapter 2) if you use them at high doses and/or over a long period of time, or at normal dosages if you are predisposed to these consequences. Some substances have greater dependency potential than others; cocaine has probably the highest. Tranquilizers and sleeping pills, however, have the greatest potential for severe and dangerous withdrawal reactions, greater even than for heroin (withdrawal from which is popularly exaggerated). This category of prescription pill—the sedative-hypnotics—includes those contemporary wonder drugs, the benzodiazepine sleeping pills and tranquilizers (Valium, Librium, Dalmane, Ativan, Serax, Xanax, etc.) which are often taken with as little concern as Alka-Seltzer. Introduced a couple of decades ago, these drugs have been touted as the most effective and safe ever known. Yet within the last few years Valium has been singled out as producing withdrawal when users suddenly stop taking it. Moreover, it has been shown that some people (the same 10-percenters with the family history) get hooked on it at clinically recommended dosages.

4. **MYTH: Valium is the most dangerous tranquilizer.**

REALITY: While it is true that in the emergency rooms tracked by the Drug Abuse Warning Network (DAWN) of the National Institute on Drug Abuse (NIDA) in more than 25 cities nationwide in 1980, and again in 1981, the number one prescription drug of abuse was diazepam (the chemical name for Valium), all the drugs in the benzodiazepine class have the same potential for trouble. They cause dependency and barbiturate-type, potentially life-threatening withdrawal symptoms. Because Valium has been the most widely prescribed benzodiazepine, and until 1982 was the most frequently prescribed of all drugs, the problems began to be noticed among Valium users and became associated by the public and doctors exclusively with that product. Almost all the tranquilizers and "light" sleeping pills in use today are in the benzodiazepine class. Doctors who switch their patients from Valium to related products, as many are doing, are only contributing to their patients' dependency problems. (See "cross-tolerance," p. 44.)

---

5. **MYTH: Alcohol is less dangerous than the drugs they sell on the street. Otherwise it wouldn't be legal.**

REALITY: Alcohol is a psychoactive drug and despite its legal status is the drug *most* dangerous to body, mind, and public safety. As *Drug Abuse, A Guide for the Primary Care Physician* parenthetically puts it: "The degree of hazard associated with drug use can be assessed in terms of (1) the immediate psychic and physical effects of the drug on the individual and (2) the consequences of continued drug use to society as a whole. (Based on these considerations, alcohol is far more hazardous than any other drug. As Gay and Way observe in *It's So Good, Don't Even Try It Once* [Englewood Cliffs, NJ: Prentice-Hall, 1972], 'in terms of incidence of use, complications from acute overdose, long-term effects on the physical and mental state of an individual, and ultimate consequences for society, there is no close second to alcohol.')"

Because alcohol is legal, we naturally assume it can't be so bad. (Alcohol is safe only in small amounts and never in combination with most drugs.) This misconception in turn leads to the worst of inadvertent consequences. Alcohol is often the factor which makes use of an otherwise safe drug lethal. Alcohol in combination with other drugs caused more injuries and deaths in the DAWN hospitals than any single substance could alone. Valium, for example, is virtually impossible to kill yourself with, one of the reasons doctors are so happy to prescribe it. In the DAWN data, however, Valium accounts for the greatest number of drug-related deaths, and 95.5 percent of the Valium-related deaths were caused by that drug in combination with others, principally alcohol.

---

6. **MYTH: The reason so many people have prescription drug problems is that doctors prescribe too much medication for pain and anxiety in hospitals and clinical practice.**

   REALITY: If anything, the opposite is true. Evidence suggests that misinformation and misconceptions about dependency and addiction are causing doctors to run scared and undermedicate for fear of causing a drug problem. This practice does a great disservice to patients, particularly those in extreme conditions. Once doctors are able, with the help of the new body of addiction research, to identify which patients are particularly at risk for drug problems, they will be able to prescribe appropriately.

7. **MYTH: Drug dependency and drug addiction are different terms for the same thing.**

   REALITY: The two are not synonymous. Dependency is the development of a physical or psychological need for a substance, with a physical or psychological reaction to the drug's removal. Addiction is a disease marked by compulsion, loss of control, and continued use despite adverse consequences. Although a person suffering from addictive disease (see page 45) will be dependent on one or more substances, someone who is dependent on, say, cocaine, is not necessarily an addict.

8. **MYTH: Drug abuse is a young people's problem. It is not common among the elderly.**

   REALITY: Drug abuse is very much a problem for the elderly. Although the over-60 segment of DAWN respondents (1981) used drugs least often to get high, they used drugs more often than any other age group to commit suicide. (Depression is the most frequent psychiatric problem reported in the elderly.) The elderly are also most at risk for severe side effects and toxic consequences of drug use because of changes in their metabolism and deterioration of organs which process and clear these drugs from the system. Pills remain in their systems much longer, increasing the drug's toxic potential. Also, the elderly cannot tolerate ordinary side effects well. Some psychoactive drugs, for instance, can cause dizziness and loss of balance; a fall by a young person may not be serious, but a fall by an elderly person can have severe, even deadly results.

9. **MYTH: You can't be addicted to a drug you've never taken.**

REALITY: Once you have a dependency or addiction problem with a drug, you will automatically have the same potential problem with all other drugs in the same class or which act similarly, whether you have taken them or not. Alcohol, for example, behaves somewhat similarly to tranquilizers and sedatives. An alcoholic who begins to take these pills (frequently upon prescription from a doctor to deal with some of the symptoms of alcoholism) will quickly become addicted to them.

10. **MYTH: Your doctor will inform you of all the risks involved in taking the medication he or she is prescribing for you.**

REALITY: Although "it is a medical duty to apprise the public of the facts concerning the extensive usage and the merits and disadvantages of these drugs" (*Introduction to Psychopharmacology*, published for doctors by the Upjohn Company), not all doctors are up on the facts—and not all of them care to share these details with their patients.

But a doctor's responsibility is only half the story. (Principles of proper prescribance are detailed in chapter 6.) As attitudes toward doctors as unquestioned authorities change, the role of personal responsibility toward one's own health and health care grows proportionately. Ultimately it's your decision whether or not to take a drug. Therefore it's your responsibility to seek information. As they say—it's your body.

2

Psychoactive Drugs and the Body: The Physical Side of Abuse

No two people react to a drug, even to a cigarette, in the same way. No two people taking the same drug arrive at drug abuse following the same route. Indeed, once drug abuse is established, the pattern is never the same for any two people taking the identical substance—Alberta takes her tranquilizers at night with a nip or two of brandy; Michael takes his in the morning with four cups of coffee.

Drug abuse is influenced by an array of physiological, genetic, pharmacological, social, psychological, environmental, economic factors—even acts of God. These variables combine to make each person's experience unique.

Drug abuse begins simply enough (or so it seems): a person and a chemical substance come together at some time and place and begin to interact.

FROM BLOOD TO BRAIN

Taken by mouth, your pill enters the bloodstream by being absorbed into the blood's plasma at any point along the gastrointestinal tract. For most drugs, an empty stomach will promote the most rapid absorption.

Once the drug is absorbed, it must be delivered by the blood to the organ or tissues where its effects are required. On its way toward the target area—the central nervous system (mostly brain but also spine)—the blood is routed first through the liver. As far as the liver is concerned, most drugs are "chemical invaders"—poisons which it must deactivate and expel from the system. Liver enzymes act at once to break down the drugs into inactive substances (metabolites), rendering them harmless and ineffective. But not all the drug is deactivated on the blood's first pass

34

through the liver (if it were, no drug would have any effect at all). The breakdown process—metabolism—occurs continously as the blood circulates.

Thus the blood delivers the active drug to your brain and the inactive metabolites are delivered by the liver back into the bloodstream. As the blood passes through the kidneys, the inactive materials are drawn out to be eliminated in the urine. The kidneys will also eliminate some of the active drug that has not yet been broken down or distributed to the brain.

The longer an active drug is in the body, the longer its good effects and bad (side) effects will continue. To increase drug effectiveness, pharmacologists have been able to design pills which can "fool" the body into delaying metabolism and excretion. For example, the action of liver enzymes on some benzodiazepines (Valium and Librium included), instead of deactivating them, transforms them into other, *more active* metabolites. This, of course, extends the medication's life span inside your body.

The kidneys, too, can be kept from removing the still active drug from the system. Most psychoactive drugs are chemically designed so that in their active state the kidneys will reabsorb them and return them to the bloodstream rather than letting them pass down into the bladder. Only when the liver has finally deactivated them completely will they be in a chemical state to be readily excreted. How long deactivation and elimination takes depends on the chemistry of the particular drug and a host of physiological and genetic factors in each individual consumer. Pharmacologists measure the active life span of each drug in terms of its *plasma half-life*, the time it takes for the blood plasma concentration of the drug to be reduced by half. Amphetamines have a half-life of 5 hours. However, if a person's urine is more than ordinarily acidic, the excretion of unmetabolized amphetamine still in the blood will be speeded up and the drug will have less effect.

Some drugs (among them phenobarbital and some other barbiturates, plus alcohol, caffeine, and nicotine) after repeated use are capable of causing a much more rapid rate of metabolism. This does not happen in everyone; scientists believe it is in part genetically determined. The half-life of phenobarbital, for example, can vary from 53 to 118 hours. A person in whom the drug is more quickly metabolized has to take more of it to get the benefit of the medication, but taking more also increases the risk of side effects and toxic effects.

Mixing certain psychoactive drugs will sometimes shorten, more frequently lengthen, their half-lives. When the half-life is lengthened, overdose becomes more likely. In the elderly, deterioration of organs involved in metabolism, principally the liver and kidneys, also extends the active life span of drugs such as diazepam. The elderly are much more at risk of accidental overdose from self-medicating or if a physician does not prescribe appropriately.

Drugs with long half-lives and drugs which are not properly cleared may accumulate and be stored in body tissues. Released into the bloodstream, they again become active until they are finally fully metabolized. This is why PCP can cause an unexpected and frequently undesired psychoactive effect long after it is taken.

ALTERING THE BRAIN'S CHEMISTRY

What happens when the drug reaches the brain is becoming known as research brings the biochemistry of the brain into focus. While antibiotics work by attacking organisms which infect the body, thus curing the condition, psychoactive drugs alter the brain's chemistry. They "cure" nothing— they simply block or encourage the receipt or delivery of certain nerve messages, changing, for example, "Ouch!" to "Whew, that's better!" or "Pass the peanut butter!" to "No thanks, I couldn't eat a thing!"

Thus psychoactive drugs offer only symptomatic relief. Once a person afflicted with schizophrenia goes off antipsychotic medication, the terrible symptoms will resume in the same way that consciousness returns when anesthesia wears off, or that anxiety and muscle spasms reappear when the effects of a tranquilizer are gone.

Psychoactive drugs affect the neurotransmitters: brain chemicals which carry the nerve impulses across synapses (gaps) from cell to cell. These neurotransmitters, which include serotonin, dopamine, acetylcholine, epinephrine (adrenaline), norepinephrine, and others which are still being discovered, act essentially to turn on or turn off, or speed up or slow down, basic functions which influence behavior. These include sleep, waking, pain, anxiety, pleasure, alertness, judgment, mood, emotion, cognition, appetite, motor activity, sexual experience, aggressivity, consciousness, and memory.

Psychoactive drugs either block the receptor sites at the other side of the synapses so that the neurotransmitters can't deliver their nerve impulse messages, or they activate the receptor sites so that the messages will have a greater impact.

Some of the psychoactive drugs seem actually to replace the brain's own neurotransmitters. There is some suggestion that they may all do this; it is known now that the molecules of the opiates (heroin for one) and the benzodiazepines (Valium, etc.) fit so snugly into neurotransmitter receptor sites that they must be pushing some endogenous chemical (one that is produced by the body) out of the way. In 1975 Scottish researchers discovered the first of a previously unknown class of neurotransmitters—called endorphins—which apparently are the body's own natural pain relievers and ecstasy makers. They are present in minute amounts and are astonishingly similar in structure to the opiate drugs.

Natural neurotransmitters similar to tranquilizers have yet to be located. But since the benzodiazepines fit like pieces of a puzzle (or keys in a lock) into specific receptor sites, scientists hypothesize that the body must produce its own tranquilizers. After all, would our genes create molecular receptors and just wait for Valium to be invented?

As we shall see, receptor sites have much to do with dependency and addiction.

DRUG ACTIONS

Psychoactive drugs are generally classed in groups by their principal action or effect on the central nervous system. (These drug groups are described in detail in section II, and it is essential to your understanding of any pill you are taking to know the group to which it belongs.)

Stimulants do just that—hype you up: cocaine, amphetamine, caffeine, nicotine.

Sedative-hypnotics slow you down and/or put you to sleep. They include the benzodiazepines (Valium, etc.) and the barbiturates (Seconal, Tuinal, phenobarbital).

Narcotic analgesics—the opiates, their derivatives, and

related drugs such as Percodan, Codeine, and Demerol—produce a different pattern and quality of sleep from that of sedative-hypnotics and relieve pain.

Antidepressants relieve the symptoms of depression and anxiety. They include Adapin, Elavil, and Tofranil.

Antipsychotics attack the symptoms of major mental illness and help control behavior. They include Thorazine, Haldol, Prolixin, and Mellaril.

More than other pharmaceuticals, psychoactive drugs seem to have a multitude of additional actions. This is because the same substances are often involved in many or all of the central nervous system's complex activities. The central nervous system not only regulates how we feel and respond and what we know, but regulates the body's other systems.

The more influence a drug has over these states and systems, the more dangerous it can be. For example, antidepressants, besides influencing mood, affect the heart and blood pressure, muscle coordination, digestion, blood sugar, sex drive, and still other body functions. Barbiturates (such as Seconal) put you to sleep and also influence your breathing. Besides suppressing appetite and stimulating wakefulness, amphetamines speed up all body systems, circulatory system included.

The more specific the action of a drug, the safer it tends to be, although no psychoactive drug is completely safe. The opiates and the benzodiazepines, which act primarily on particular receptor sites in certain areas of the brain only, have less influence over multiple body systems and are considered relatively safe (when used alone and under controlled conditions). They can produce well defined toxic effects but have a wide therapeutic ratio.

In future, the more scientists discover about exactly which receptors are responsible for what, the more they will be able to design drugs whose molecules are targeted to those sites only. The result will be that you will be able to get the benefit of the medication without having to pay for it in uncomfortable and sometimes dangerous side effects. Another result will be, possibly, that the pills you take to relieve pain will not also get you high.

SIDE EFFECTS AND TOXIC EFFECTS

So far, even the drugs with the most specific action have additional effects. The extra effects and actions of a drug are called its side effects. They result either from the additional pharmacological actions of the drug or from the strength of the dose. Drowsiness, for example, is a common side effect of many psychoactive drugs; so is dry mouth, and so is getting high.

Side effects, detailed for each drug or drug group in section II, range from tiredness to increased or decreased sex drive to rapid heart rate to insomnia—and to feelings of euphoria, peace, joy, fearlessness, competence, happiness—depending on the drug. Obviously, the side effects are often what a drug is taken for, nonmedically speaking.

Toxic or adverse effects are the severest side effects. This is what nobody wants—for the substance to begin to act like poison to mind and body systems.

Side effects (including the high) often disappear if the drug is taken continuously. Through the phenomenon of tolerance, your body works to return to a state of equilibrium in the presence of the drug.

Generally, the degree of side effects, from mild to toxic, is related to the potency of the dose as well as to how long the drug is continuously in your body. This dose relationship is an avenue of abuse in recreational drug use: the higher the dose, the greater the high, the greater the risk of toxic effects. Alcohol causes the worst side effects of all, particularly on the brain and on the organs which have to metabolize it, liver, pancreas, and kidneys. Sometimes the toxic effect of a drug is the opposite of what you take it for: instead of peace, anxiety; instead of a clear mind, confusion, even psychosis; instead of relaxation, convulsions.

Prescription drug dosages are carefully developed and courses of therapy recommended to achieve maximum desired effects and minimum adverse ones. Self-medicating interferes with that—yet another reason why "harmless" prescription drugs become unsafe in nonprofessional hands.

Needless to say, drugs that cannot legally be prescribed, such as heroin and marijuana, have no recommended dosages. And none of the illicit drugs, lookalikes included, are regulated for uniformity, purity, or quality as are the Rx's. The risk of unpredictable overdose on the street is far greater for these reasons.

DEPENDENCY

Dependency is an adverse effect of all psychoactive drugs—even the "mild" ones. Dependency will happen to anybody at a high enough and/or long enough dosage. Some drugs have a greater dependency potential than others (see the table on p. 51). For example, cigarettes have an estimated 80 percent potential: eight out of every ten persons who begin to smoke will develop a habit. For marijuana, also smoked, the rate is only 3 to 6 percent, according to some estimates.

And some people have a higher dependency potential—among them the ten-percenters with the family history, who will develop dependencies at lower dosages.

Dependency is a curious thing. For reasons that remain unclear, after repeated, usually high-dose exposure to these substances, the body develops a need for them—not necessarily for the special effect the drug provides, but rather to feel normal. This spells trouble, for at this point the drug's role in your life has changed from something incidental to something fundamental. To food, clothing, and shelter, add drug. Unless tolerance is present, however, the need for the drug may not be apparent until you try to go off it.

Physical Dependency and Withdrawal

There are two kinds of dependency: physical (also called chemical) and psychological. In physical dependency the substance becomes biochemically necessary for body cells to function normally. The sedative-hypnotics and narcotic-analgesics produce physical dependency. The stimulants are believed to cause a primarily psychological or mixed physical/psychological dependency pattern.

The mechanism of physical dependency may have to do with the neurotransmitters and their receptor sites. One theory suggests that when opiates are introduced into the system, they at first supplement or stimulate the natural neurotransmitter systems (in this case the endorphins); hence the relief of pain or the euphoria. Ultimately, however, this overstimulation or excessive amount of substance causes a shutdown of the natural system. The opiate—say, heroin—now replaces the normal substance.

But when the drug is suddenly removed, the cells cannot function normally until the body becomes able to produce or use its own biochemicals properly. Until then there is the withdrawal period or abstinence syndrome, with symptoms varying in onset and duration for each drug.

The narcotics user is not the only true addict, nor is narcotics withdrawal the worst of all possible nightmares. The sedative-hypnotic drugs and alcohol have far greater potential for precipitating life-threatening seizures, while withdrawal from heroin is rather like a bad case of the flu.

Withdrawal from a drug, the benzodiazepines in particular, may trigger an intense return of the symptoms (such as anxiety) for which the drug was originally taken. Current research indicates that the benzodiazepines may cause a second, more protracted withdrawal phase following the acute phase in the susceptible ten-percenters.

Only continued use of the substance will prevent the abstinence syndrome or stop it once it has started—which explains in good measure why some of the nicest folks will continue to abuse drugs even in the presence of clear health hazards.

Psychological Dependency and Withdrawal

In psychological dependency the cells have no need for the drug in order to continue to function, but the psyche does. Here, withdrawal is primarily an emotional experience. Cocaine and speed produce powerful psychological dependencies. Stopping, especially abruptly, can cause horrible depression, sense of helplessness, severe exhaustion, and inability to function. This is not a physiological crisis, but it is still a crisis. According to Shana Alexander, in her book *Very Much a Lady: The Untold Story of Jean Harris and Dr. Herman Tarnower*, the private-school headmistress was in withdrawal from a ten-year Desoxyn habit and was "coming unglued" when she shot the Scarsdale Diet doctor in 1980.

In psychological dependency, the psyche becomes reliant on a drug for equilibrium. This is not only a human phenomenon. Monkeys and rats in experimental settings will go for the "reward" that cocaine provides. The more they get of it, the more they want it and the more uncomfortable they become without it; the substance becomes essential to their psychological "steady state." Psychologists use the term "reinforcement" to describe this learning process.

Reinforcement can lead to another function of psychological dependency, "state-dependent learning." Once Harvey, the blocked screenwriter in the previous chapter, became dependent on amphetamine, he could no longer write without it. And poor Tom—listen to what happened to his sex life. He was a perfectly normal 24-year-old guy who discovered that small amounts of amphetamine and cocaine would jazz up his sex life. After a while, sex and stimulants always went together; he started smoking cocaine freebase and injecting speed (and taking tranquilizers to come down). And suddenly poor Tom could get an erection no more. He went off all drugs—which wasn't easy after all that time—but his predrug sexual functioning didn't return. He had learned to associate sex with being stoned—state-dependent learning—and now, in psychotherapy, he had to relearn how to function in a different state.

It's as if Pavlov's dog, having learned to salivate at the sound of a bell, could no longer salivate without it.

Mixed Dependencies

People who have used a drug recreationally to the point of physical dependency are almost always psychologically dependent on it as well. It is relatively simple to detoxify heroin addicts. It is another matter to keep them off the stuff, because, particularly after a long habit, their life-style has become so conditioned to heroin's effects and to other users that they are at sea without their habit.

Cigarettes are an example of a mixed dependency pattern. Nicotine is a minor central nervous system stimulant which is only very mildly physically addicting; physical withdrawal is over in the first couple of days. The rest of the agony is psychological (similar to cocaine withdrawal) and can last for months; some people report sudden cravings years later.

When physical dependency results from medical use, psychological dependency may not be present. It depends on how much the drug has become associated with normal psychological functioning. Hospitalized patients who have become physically dependent on narcotics used to treat painful conditions may not even realize it if the medication is gradually removed before they are released to go home.

TOLERANCE

Tolerance is a state in which the same dosage of a drug no longer achieves the required or desired effect. It is often a symptom of physical or psychological dependency—frequently the first clear sign that it is developing. (It is, however, possible to become dependent on a drug without acquiring tolerance; then, in some cases of physical dependency, withdrawal may be the primary sign.) Here you've been taking your nightly 15 milligrams of, for example, Dalmane for two weeks to get to sleep and now it doesn't work. The natural response—particularly among those who dose themselves—is to take 30 milligrams. But eventually a state of tolerance is reached again; the drug is less effective or you need more.

The only way to stop the buildup of tolerance once it has started is to stop taking the drug (see chapter 4 for tips on stopping, and also check the drug out in section II). Lower doses will again be effective after a period of abstinence (generally related to the level of tolerance that has been built). But again, with repeated use tolerance will begin to build.

Tolerance arises out of the same mechanism which accounts for the disappearance of side effects. The body works, as always, to reestablish equilibrium, by metabolizing the drug faster and getting rid of it before it can have an effect, or by altering receptor sensitivity so that the effect is lessened. Degree or rate of acquired tolerance is probably influenced by genetic factors—as well as by repeated drug use at high dosage.

Tolerance gives birth to the "monkey on your back"—the habit that has to be fed in greater and greater quantities. Narcotics addicts with large habits are not getting more stoned than those with more moderate habits; on the contrary, they require huge amounts to feel normal, and to get just a little high.

Tolerance is associated with most patterns of drug abuse and with all patterns of addiction. And, as its name implies, as tolerance develops your body can accept more of the drug with less actual or apparent ill effect. What gives a long-time narcotics user a so-so buzz would kill a newer user (which is how many heroin deaths occur). But tolerance does not build to all effects; this can lead to false confidence (always the biggest trap of drug abuse) about a drug's safety among long-time users. Sedative-hypnotic tolerance, for example, builds to the sleep-inducing and calming aspects, but not completely, and not, eventually, to the lethal aspects. Somebody who has been taking barbiturates for years to get to sleep may finally increase the dose one more small fraction—and die.

Tolerance to amphetamines can occur with the high, appetite suppression, and effects on blood pressure and heartbeat; however, the risk of psychosis continues to increase with the dosage.

Virtually complete narcotic-analgesic tolerance occurs to the pain-killing, intoxicating, and calming effects. Research suggests that under laboratory conditions, tolerance to even the lethal effects may be possible. But in practice, when drugs such as heroin, China white, and "loads" are obtained from street sources, the quality and purity are so low or so unpredictable that tolerance does not build sufficiently to protect the user; death is possible from overdose even for long-time users. Also, narcotics high in purity are often responsible for deaths among those who are accustomed to drugs cut with other substances.

In short courses of treatment at recommended clinical dosages, tolerance to medical drugs is unlikely to occur—except among the susceptible ten-percenters. *Tolerance should be a red flag to both doctor and patient.* If the drug is discontinued, further problems with tolerance can be avoided.

Cross-Tolerance

Once you have acquired tolerance to a psychoactive drug, you will have acquired equivalent tolerance to other, related drugs. Cross-tolerance tends to develop among drugs in the same class, which is one reason why drugs of the same class have been grouped together in section II. If your dentist has been prescribing increasing doses of Darvon, say, for the three months you've been enduring root canal work, and he then switches you to codeine, you'll need just as much of it and receive as little effect— because the two drugs are both narcotic-analgesic. It is also pointless to switch patients with Valium problems to another benzodiazepine tranquilizer.

Drugs from different classes are cross-tolerant if they achieve the same effect, regardless of chemical structure. This means that problems like pain, anxiety, and sleeplessness become extremely difficult to treat in the presence of cross-tolerance. Forty-six-year-old Tony G. had been a narcotics addict so long he couldn't remember, he confessed to a nurse at the hospital where he was brought by ambulance after a motorcycle accident. He had broken two vertebrae in his neck and was in severe pain. But he had built such a degree of cross-tolerance to narcotic pain-killers that there was little the doctors could do to ease his suffering.

Those who have built a tolerance to alcohol will be cross-tolerant to all sedative-hypnotics, possibly to certain of the narcotic-analgesics, and to some gas anesthesias, all of which have effects similar to alcohol's on the central nervous system. To achieve an effect from drugs, an alcoholic may have to be exposed to dangerously high doses.

ADDICTION

Addiction is a disease and as such it differs from other drug abuse problems. It too features tolerance to increased dosage and physical and/or psychological dependency, but is also marked by compulsion and loss of control despite the consequences. The addict may have decided to have just one drink or just one "line" of cocaine, but will be compelled to continue, frequently until the supply is finished. The pattern will be repeated time after time, despite the loss of employment, family, friends, health, and self-respect.

An abuser who is not an addict may experience equally strong desire but will be able to control the drug when the consequences begin to get out of hand and the resolve to stop or cut back is made. Linda D., for example, got into a cocaine habit along with most of her affluent young professional friends. Just the thought of cocaine would trigger a craving for it. But because she found herself *always* thinking about it, and always doing it, she began to regret her lack of control, especially when she began to experience severe morning-after depressions. She decided she had better cut down on her use. Linda instituted a once-a-week, three-lines-maximum rule. In spite of this, for the first couple of weeks she snorted three or four days each, four or five lines. But at least it wasn't every day anymore, and after about a month she was able to level off at once or twice a week. Some weeks she could go without it entirely.

An addict might be able to restrict the days of use (there are plenty of weekend or periodic alcoholics) but not the amount each time. Once the drug triggers the compulsion, attempts to control behavior are useless. For an addict, the only way out is to prevent the compulsion. And the only way to do that is to remain drug-free. *Controlled use may be possible with other patterns of abuse, but never with addiction.*

Addiction is a chronic, relapsing disease which will reappear as soon as the substance is reintroduced—no matter how long the addict has been drug-free. And it is potentially fatal.

The 10 Percent Factor

Anyone can become addicted, but the tendency toward addiction appears to have a strong genetic basis. As mentioned earlier, research conducted throughout the last decade reveals that fully 10 percent of the population has a psychobiological predisposition to drug dependency and addiction. In some people, the disease will become manifest the very first time the triggering substance is used (see the story of Frank Jr. below); in these people, genes are the determining factors. For most of the predisposed population, however, the disease seems to arise out of an interaction of genetic and behavioral/environmental factors. (A small percentage of addicts acquire the disease without demonstrating a predisposition; for them behavioral/environmental factors are sufficient to cause the addiction; see below.)

In these respects, addiction is like diabetes, which may be caused by 1) genetic factors only, accounting for the early-onset type; 2) genetic predisposition plus obesity (a behavioral/environmental factor); or 3) obesity alone.

Within addict recovery groups, it is not uncommon to find as many as ninety percent with a family history of alcohol or drug abuse. Frank and Irene have been members of Alcoholics Anonymous for 25 years. Both come from families with serious drinking problems. They have one son, Frank Jr., who is also an alcoholic. His disease became manifest when he was fifteen and accepted a vodka and orange juice at a party. Then he asked for another, and another, and another—he had become immediately compulsive—until, long before the party ended, he blacked out. Frank Jr. was an addict. To avoid the course of the disease, his only choice was to stay away from alcohol (and other drugs—see cross-addiction, p. 48) entirely.

The immediate onset of his symptoms and the absence of environmental triggers (explained in the following chapter) indicated to addiction specialists that Frank Jr.'s addiction was probably of the purely genetic type. Others, however, may require repeated exposure to high-addiction-potential drugs to trigger their predisposition.

Drugs with High Addiction Potential

Some drugs have greater potential for compulsive use and thus are more likely to trigger addiction, just as ice cream is more likely than a hunk of liver to trigger a binge in a compulsive eater. They have a quick, powerful onset of action and probably stimulate the receptor sites strongly. (Onset of action is itself an important variable of drug abuse.) They include the narcotic-analgesics, the short-acting barbiturates (such as amobarbital, pentobarbital, and secobarbital), and cocaine.

A man in his mid-twenties who had been taking Dilantin and phenobarbital (the latter a slow-acting barbiturate) for years for a seizure disorder, exhibited an immediate compulsion when Seconal (secobarbital) was prescribed for insomnia related to work-related stress. He was soon taking so many Seconals—five to ten a day—that he cracked up his car and killed two people. It turned out he had a family history of alcoholism; it took the faster-acting barbiturate to trigger his predisposition. After he was detoxified from Seconal, his Dilantin/phenobarbital did not spark the compulsion. (He was acquitted in the legal action brought against him, his lawyer proving that he had suffered an unavoidable drug reaction.)

Unfortunately, predisposed individuals are not necessarily protected from drugs with lower potential, generally those which pack less of a wallop, like tranquilizers. With a family history, you are far more likely to be hypersensitive to *all* psychoactive substances. Abruptly stopping even small amounts of a drug, tranquilizers included, may precipitate acute withdrawal. With benzodiazepine use you may be uniquely at risk of a second, prolonged withdrawal phase following the acute phase.

Why this hypersensitivity occurs is not fully understood. Addicts and predisposed individuals in general appear to process psychoactive drugs differently, both in the liver and at the neurotransmitter-receptor site level.

Cross-Addiction

Addiction to any psychoactive substance greatly increases the risk of rapid addiction to other drugs, including those with low addiction potential. Cross-addiction, like cross-tolerance, occurs with drugs that act similarly, like sedatives and alcohol. Many alcoholics become "prescription junkies" when their physicians, apparently unaware of the risk of cross-addiction, prescribe tranquilizers or other sedatives to offset alcoholic shakiness and similar symptoms.

Cross-addiction can occur even after prolonged abstinence from the primary drug, and what's worse, the new addiction will reactivate the craving for the old one.

The cross-addiction process may be related to the neurotransmitter receptor sites. Alcohol appears to alter them, perhaps making the sites more sensitive to the "message"; a whisper, so to speak, comes across as a shout, with consequent biological and behavioral overreaction. Once the neurotransmitter-receptor mechanism is damaged, even a "weaker" similar drug will affect the transmission of nerve-cell messages in the same inappropriate way.

Obviously, it is essential that addicts be medicated differently from nonaddicts (see chapter 6).

Addiction with No Family History

Like the diabetic who develops the disease by way of obesity without heredity, some abusers move into addiction purely by way of compulsive, continuous drug use. Anybody will become an addict to some drugs after long enough use at high enough doses. The triggers are emotional and environmental. An estimated 20 percent of GIs in Vietnam became addicted to heroin—a much higher incidence than in the armed services before or since. Upon their return, over 90 percent were able to give up heroin.

Once it is established, drug addiction, with or without predisposition, follows a similar course of escalating tolerance, decreasing controls, physical and mental anguish, and increased risk of death from overdose, complications, or suicide.

Drug Addiction and Other Compulsions

Some researchers feel that all compulsive behavior, including nonstop videogame playing, food binging, chain smoking, gambling—even compulsive jogging—are different manifestations of one addictive phenomenon. Whether family history plays a part is not known; this is a relatively new line of research that has not produced conclusive data. It has long been known, however, that many drug addicts are compulsive with other substances and activities. Many a heroin addict is pleased as Punch to be off narcotics—while smoking five packs a day and stuffed to the ears with carbohydrates. Others take up jogging during recovery and find they increase their mileage, despite frequent injuries, to achieve the "runner's high." Some even report withdrawal symptoms when they are forced to stop running. (Recent research suggests that prolonged exercise may trigger the endorphins, the endogenous opiatelike neurotransmitters, accounting for the high.) Nondrug alternatives for the management of symptoms such as anxiety are very important for individuals with addictive disease.

COMBINING PSYCHOACTIVE DRUGS

Drug abuse statistics indicate that half of the people who end up in the emergency room and two-thirds of those in the morgue arrive courtesy of a combination of drugs. The overwhelming majority combine their drugs with alcohol.

Alcohol is poison with other psychoactive substances. It is a potentiator—it makes other drugs much more potent in all their effects, including intoxicating and lethal ones. This begins in the liver, where alcohol and sedative drugs compete for the same metabolic enzymes, thus slowing the ordinary deactivation and elimination process and powerfully extending the sedative's effects and life span. Taken along with other drugs which depress, or slow, the system, alcohol can be the killing factor, triggering respiratory failure. Many accidental sleeping-pill deaths are caused by a reasonable dose of medication plus alcohol, which may remain active in the system from a party earlier that evening.

In alcoholics and others who have a long history of alcohol use in large quantities, a diseased liver may further potentiate the effects of drugs by metabolizing them less efficiently.

Other drugs may also interact with each other and cause problems. In the 1981 DAWN emergency room statistics, the most frequently reported combinations (excluding alcohol) were morphine/cocaine, heroin/cocaine, Quāālude/Valium, Dalmane/Valium, and cocaine/Valium. Quāālude/Valium and Dalmane/Valium are both central nervous system depressant combinations which, like alcohol/sedatives, will multiply the risk of respiratory failure and coma.

Karen Quinlan remains in a coma in New Jersey after her life supports were removed in a landmark life-support case in 1974. Although the cause of her condition has not been conclusively established, she was reported to have taken a sedative-hypnotic and alcohol that fateful night. Just for fun, her friends said, and not "too much" of either.

Stimulant-depressant combinations like heroin/morphine plus cocaine and cocaine/Valium are often used to get a particular quality of intoxication or to counteract each other's effects or side effects ("downers" to bring a person off the racing effects of "uppers" in order, perhaps, to get some sleep or calm the shakes). Repeatedly combining drugs may promote mixed dependencies, cross-addictions, and severe withdrawal crises, not to mention the multiple effects on the brain and body.

Patients receiving different drugs from different specialists are at risk. If your dentist prescribes codeine for root canal pain, your psychiatrist gives you Placidyl to help break an insomnia cycle, and your orthopedist orders Valium for your bad back, don't just stand there—inform each of them of the other drugs you are taking. Hospitalized patients being seen by many specialists (for example, heart surgeon and cardiologist for a coronary bypass, neurologist and gastroenterologist for postsurgical complications) should make a point of asking the nurses to keep track of all medications and to intervene, if necessary, on their behalf.

DRUG ABUSE RISKS BY DRUG CLASS

	Primary Nature of Dependency	Dependency Potential	Risk of Organ Damage and/or Death	Risk of Severe Social/ Economic Consequences	Risk of Severe and/or Long-Lasting Mental/ Behavioral Change
Stimulants	psychological	high	moderate	moderate to high	moderate to high
Barbiturates	physical	moderate to high	moderate to high	moderate to high	low
Benzodiazepines	physical	low	low	low	low
Narcotic analgesics	physical	high	low	high	low to moderate
Alcohol	physical	moderate	high	high	high
Cannabinoids (Marijuana)	psychological	low to moderate	low	low to moderate	low
Cigarettes	physical/ psychological	high	high	low	low
Mixed drug classes	physical/ psychological	high	high	high	high

A hospital can turn out to be a dangerous place for those of you who are susceptible ten-percenters—the place where you are introduced to the high-potential drug to which you will become addicted. Doctors are more likely to prescribe more powerful drugs in a hospital, because the patient can be watched there. A week's worth of morphine or Seconal may trigger your predisposition.

3
Drugs and Your Lifestyle: The Psychological Side of Abuse

You are a feeling, thinking, acting human being. You are exposed to a drug within a given environment:

• the circumstances of your life;
• your past and your foreseeable future;
• the pressures you are under;
• how you respond to stress;
• who your friends are;
• what your job is;
• how much money you have;
• where or when you take your drugs;
• your family life;
• your state of mind;
• the state of the economy;
• your health.

These have as much to do with your choosing a drug and becoming a user, abuser, or addict as your genes and how the drug acts inside your body. Even for a drug addict with a strong psychobiological predisposition, some outside factor must trigger it. The drug itself is the first outside factor—it comes from the environment. How does it happen that you take the drug? The following case history illustrates all too well how the environment can provide the determining factors.

Marianne is an addict. You'd never know it to look at her. She's a lawyer and holds a prestigious government job in a large northeastern city. She's 27 and comes from an upper-class New England family—prep schools and Ivy League all the way. Marianne's mother drank large amounts of alcohol daily at the social events which were her principal occupation. Like many children of problem drinkers, Marianne rarely drank. Her mother's drinking and often abusive behavior disgusted her. Throughout her schooling, Marianne wasn't exposed to alcohol much, since she was as intent on her studies as her mother was on socializing. Her city government job exposed her to many political events and business lunches where she was known as a teetotaler.

During a tennis game one day, Marianne twisted around suddenly. Sharp, insistent pain began the next day. She saw a doctor who prescribed Valium for muscle spasm and first Tylenol with codeine, then SK-65 (a generic Darvon preparation), and ultimately Percodan, for the pain. But the pain did not substantially subside and the doctor advised that Marianne stay in bed. At home she began taking steadily increasing doses of Percodan, along with the Tylenol/codeine and the SK-65 that remained from the initial prescriptions, plus the Valium. Mostly she watched TV and drifted. When Marianne phoned her doctor for more Percodan and Valium, the doctor obliged, even though both prescriptions should have lasted longer.

Marianne was able to go back to her job when the time came, but continued to be in pain—that, or she wanted to keep taking the pills, even she wasn't sure anymore. When her doctor at last became reluctant to prescribe, Marianne stole several sheets off the prescription pad and wrote her own prescriptions, forging the doctor's signature. It could have meant the end of her career, even jail, had Marianne been found out. She wasn't—but her City Hall colleagues had started to whisper about her "drunkenness," assuming she must be a closet alcoholic. What other explanation could there be for her dull-witted, uncoordinated, glassy-eyed demeanor? And it was no secret that she wasn't doing her work. She began to call in sick one, sometimes two days a week.

Finally, her commissioner called her in and asked if she would like to take a leave of absence. Without having to explain, Marianne accepted with relief. She wanted out of this horrible thing. She was so ashamed that she wouldn't even seek help in her own city; she flew all the way to the West Coast for treatment.

Marianne's story illustrates several personal and environmental variables, among them availability, source, attitude, setting, and health. The drugs that sparked Marianne's addiction were not available in her normal environment. They become *available*, however, when she was injured (*health*), through her doctor (the *source*). Marianne would have refused alcohol under any circumstances, but her *attitude* toward prescription drugs was open and accepting. Perhaps the crucial variable for Marianne was the *setting*. Had she been at work rather than lying in bed bored with all those pills around, she probably would have exercised her usual rather rigid controls. She might have been able to fight the taste for the drugs that she was rapidly developing and to head off the compulsion which, once in motion, nearly led her to self-destruct.

ATTITUDES

Attitudes—personal and those of society at large—strongly influence the choice of substances and shape the abuse pattern. The dominant attitude in America today is that no self-respecting person would try heroin—which keeps many a self-respecting person away from it, despite a curiosity about what the drug might be like. Those who develop a heroin habit, however, must contend with society's attitudes toward them and live, if the habit is known, as deviants.

And attitudes toward legal substances as one thing, illegal substances as another, have led to the virtual epidemic of prescription drug abuse we are contending with today.

Attitudes make it easiest to choose alcohol. Even the overt drunk is often accepted and tenderly tolerated, as witness the frequency of comic sketches about lovable drunks on TV or in the movies.

AVAILABILITY, PREFERENCE, AND PRICE

Alcohol, cigarettes, prescription drugs, and marijuana are the principal drugs of abuse today because they are available almost everywhere.

A 67-year-old grandfather was astonished to discover how simple it was to obtain marijuana. He was receiving chemotherapy following removal of a cancerous lung. Oncologists at the teaching hospital where he was being treated recommended that he smoke or eat marijuana before each treatment to quell the disabling and discouraging nausea.

But they said they could not prescribe it for him, since even medical use of marijuana was forbidden in that state. The man called his son, a marijuana smoker, in the Midwest and asked uneasily if he could bring a supply when he came to visit in a few weeks. The son said he would, but suggested that in the meantime it would be easy enough for his father to obtain some on his own. "Me? How? I don't know any dope pushers," said the father. The son laughed and suggested that he ask any of his friends who had children living nearby if they could get some for him. After some hesitation, the father did as his son suggested. He "scored" on his first call. The daughter and son-in-law of his next-door neighbor were at his house within the hour with a gift of marijuana.

The availability of narcotics to doctors and nurses, combined with the high stress of their occupations, has resulted in a serious incidence of drug abuse within the medical profession. According to a study by S. E. D. Shortt, reported in 1979 in the *Canadian Medical Association Journal*, physicians misuse drugs twice as much as others on the same social level. Physicians who are "impaired" by drugs may go on to make dangerous drugs inappropriately available to patients.

But not all doctors or nurses who are tempted to shoot up with Demerol like its effects. Not all the kids who experiment with heroin like what it does to them; most don't. Preference, therefore, is a key factor influencing which drug or drugs become a habit.

And not all those exposed to Quaalude, for one, can afford or are willing to pay the going street rate (about $20 per pill). Alcohol is cheaper.

SOURCE

Harvey, the screenwriter with writer's block mentioned in chapter 1, had no strictures against taking his wife's diet pills to help him work, but he wouldn't purchase them from an illegal source, even though a fresh supply would have helped him complete the screenplay. For him, therefore, source was the key variable in his abuse pattern.

Similarly, many people who go from doctor to doctor to get pills wouldn't think of approaching a less legitimate source—even though some doctors who dispense prescriptions with relative ease are "script doctors," dispensing prescriptions for money, which is illegal. Getting their drugs from doctors helps these users rationalize their drug habits.

If the doctor is prescribing for a legitimate condition (anxiety or sleeplessness), the source may account for unwitting abuse.

OCCUPATION

What you do for a living determines the nature of your on-the-job pressures and may strongly influence which drug or drugs are introduced into your environment.

Many psychoactive drugs, perhaps all of them, can help break through the inhibitions suffered by many creative artists. For performing artists, drugs (among them Inderal, prescribed for high blood pressure) can ease the fear of having to go out there and do it. Entertainers such as rock groups often share their drugs prior to performances, or at least provide an environment in which drug use and abuse are readily understood and accepted.

In certain professional sports, notably football and basketball, drug taking is often an unofficial part of the job. One former professional football team physician, Arnold Mandell, says that before 1972 National Football League team physicians could write blanket presciptions for bulk purchases of amphetamines. NFL policy, however, prevented this practice after 1972. High doses were used mostly by linemen to promote aggressiveness and analgesia (painlessness) without the sedative effect of narcotics. Dr. Mandell reports the case of a defensive lineman who was suffering from intermittent impotence and marital problems—his wife was sure he was being unfaithful. When Dr. Mandell traced the impotence to his amphetamine use, the player was eager to cut down on the pills. "But this affected his playing and led to his being benched," reported Mandell.

While illicit use of stimulants—cocaine—is now the greater "scandal" in the football (and baseball and basketball) world, narcotic pain medication is routinely and legally dispensed for players' all-in-a-day's-work injuries.

In any occupation where drug taking is seen as part of the job, there is a higher probability that addiction will be triggered in anyone with a predisposition.

GROUP PRESSURE

Some authorities feel that peer pressure is the prime variable for many abusers. Use of a drug is often a means of ritual acceptance. Children, who are particularly vulnerable to peer pressure, often force themselves to continue a drug whose effects are unpleasant at first—whether cigarettes, alcohol, hallucinogens, or heroin.

Group pressure is hardly restricted to children, of course. An East Coast bridge and tunnel worker reports that her first day on the job in an apprentice position, she found that all her coworkers as well as their supervisor (all men) stopped work frequently to smoke marijuana. While she was no stranger to marijuana, she did not care to be stoned while working. But when the joint was passed to her she took it, because she felt the dangers of being excluded were worse. Despite repeated requests, she was not able to transfer to another tunnel for nine months. Now, though she no longer smokes on the job, her at-home use is much higher than it was before.

The group can determine attitudes, drug availability, and therefore consequences. In the entertainment and TV news industry, for example, cocaine use is open, accepted, and ritualized. It is also expensive, and the financial consequences to someone who develops a habit and can't afford it can be devastating.

Group pressure may be the determining factor in return to drug abuse and addiction. Drug users generally hang out with people who also use; the group as a whole often feels threatened when one of its members attempts to quit. Bill P. told his friends he was not going to take a drink that night. But at the party they went to Bill was so frequently offered a drink by these same friends—"Come on, Bill, *one* can't hurt you"—that he gave up and gave in. He couldn't stop at just one, and once more he ended up drunk.

The only choice for many people who want to give up drugs is to give up their friends too, which is too big a sacrifice for most people to endure. This is one reason why support and identification groups, described in the following chapter, are often the best places for abusers to turn for help.

SETTING

It seems a small point, but the setting—the place where you take the drug or where you are while intoxicated—can spell the difference between use and disastrous abuse. Death on the highways is all too frequently caused by this factor—driving a car while intoxicated. Likewise, a sleeping pill taken at bedtime is appropriate use, but a sleeping pill taken before operating a chainsaw will surely lead to abuse. We saw that lawyer Marianne, who gobbled her drugs while home from work and bored, might have avoided addiction in any other setting.

STRESS

Drug taking is more attractive when the environment is stressful and restricted: in times of economic difficulty, when segments of the society are dislocated and isolated, or where the miseries of daily life are high.

Mrs. S. was 59 when she began to suspect her husband was seeing a much younger woman. Mrs. S. had raised three children, all now away from home. Wife and mother had been her role in life. She had never worked; years before, her husband had talked her out of it. She had no money of her own and had never lived alone.

Mrs. S. was afraid to confront her husband, afraid to confront the truth. She let him get away with his ridiculous excuses—he said he'd joined a bowling league, he who'd never bowled in his life. When she developed problems staying asleep, her doctor prescribed Restoril. She began to mix herself a cocktail or two around nightfall, the time when ordinarily she would be fixing her husband's dinner. Mrs. S. discovered that Restoril and a martini substantially alleviated her extreme anxiety and feelings of impending doom. Her husband commented that she seemed in a better mood. But the Restoril no longer worked to keep her asleep. The doctor switched her to Seconal, a two-week supply with one refill, cautioning her not to mix it with alcohol. For a while she didn't mix them, or so she thought. She was taking the powerful Seconal at night at twice the prescribed dosage, and beginning to drink earlier in the day, still drifting from the medication. Her husband called her behavior disgusting; that night he didn't come home at all. Mrs. S. drank late into the night. When she decided to drag herself from the couch into the bedroom and go to sleep, she reached for her Seconals—or had she taken them already? Mrs. S. was too loaded to remember. She took more. Her daughter found her in the morning in a coma. Emergency measures saved her. Her husband left her and moved in with his stewardess friend. Mrs. S. is living temporarily with her daughter.

FAMILY AND SUPPORT SYSTEMS

The nature of a person's support system in times of trouble can be the most significant drug abuse variable. Major trauma—a death, breakup, rape, job loss, accident—frequently precedes the onset of drug abuse. Where drugs may have been used to cure symptoms or for a measure of enjoyment, following the trauma they become an outlet or an avenue of escape if there appears to be nowhere else to turn. Mrs. S., who had never abused anything except maybe coffee, could hardly turn to her husband in her distress, and she had not yet developed a support system among her children.

Traditionally, the family has been the primary support system. Family disintegration or difficulties are a major deciding factor in drug abuse. Parents whose children have lost control with drugs may slip into a drug problem themselves—often with the tranquilizers they turn to for their anxiety. Isolation and rejection from the family are among the many problems of the aging, who are anything but immune to drug abuse. Emergency room DAWN data show that it is people over 60 who abuse drugs the most—in order to kill themselves. (The 10–17 age group is right behind them).

Lack of family support systems for children can contribute to their use of drugs in later life, particularly children who are physically, psychologically, or sexually abused.

EMOTIONAL AND PSYCHOLOGICAL FACTORS

An "addictive personality" has long been considered sufficient to explain why someone develops a drug abuse problem. Such a personality has never been found to exist, however. Studies comparing addicts to nonaddicted drug users have never revealed any significant difference in types of psychological problems or personality traits.

Some researchers and drug treatment counselors believe that underlying depression is the psychological factor that contributes most significantly to the choice and continued use of drugs at a given time; psychoactive drugs do alter mood, and thus the state of mind of the user is an important variable. Other psychological variables are degree of stress and reaction to trauma, tendencies toward compulsive or impulsive behavior, low self-esteem (this, say some, is especially significant among children), tolerance for deviance, low frustration tolerance, and suppressed rage. A small percentage of individuals that develop multiple or polydrug problems may have major physiological problems such as a manic-depressive disorder that they are self-medicating with multiple drugs of abuse.

HEALTH

Your state of mental and physical health dictates which prescription substances you are likely to have around and how well you can tolerate their effects. Most prescription drug abuse starts with a legitimate prescription for *something*.

It's hard to say which ruined Fred's life—his back condition or the drug addiction that developed soon after the operation to correct his slipped disk 25 years ago. He took narcotics for the pain, the dosage promptly escalated, and Fred was hooked. Doctors were willing to prescribe whatever analgesic he requested through the years. He took so many pain killers containing phenacetin that he went into kidney failure. The dialysis treatments he had to endure so upset him that doctors began to prescribe the antipsychotic Thorazine. Fred isn't yet 60, but he hasn't held a job in years. He hasn't been a husband to his wife or a father to his children. And of course, it's impossible by now to treat his pain. Nobody treated it in the first place. They just fed his habit.

PATTERNS OF ABUSE

With health factors we return full circle to the pill and the body.The drug, the body, the person, the environment, all the factors conspire to start the process of drug abuse, and all combine to keep it going or to help establish control over it. If it continues, a pattern of abuse emerges that is shaped more and more by the drug or drugs taken. As shown in the table on page 51, and discussed in the previous chapter, each of the major drug groups has its pattern—no two are alike—with its risks and demands and unavoidable realities. Someone with a sedative habit is going to have to adjust his or her job performance to a lower level of alertness. (But will the employer accommodate such an adjustment?) With a firmly fixed narcotics habit, lying and dissembling loom large because of the general disapproval with which these drugs are viewed. Cocaine users may have to exercise extraordinary control to avoid the insistent attraction of this drug. Physical deterioration and unavoidable withdrawal will shape the alcoholic's existence as the years go by.

Thus life begins to accommodate itself to the substance, and not the other way around.

4
How to Know if You Have a Drug Problem

Do you have a problem with drugs? Is your drug abuse a single episode or a repeated pattern that seriously interferes with your health or your economic or social functioning? If you take drugs for whatever reason and difficulties are beginning to crop up, you probably do have a drug problem, even if the connection is not yet apparent or you just don't want to see it.

SYMPTOM NUMBER ONE: DEFENSIVENESS AND DENIAL

Ironically, the more developed and deeply ingrained the pattern of drug use, the harder it may be to see a serious potential problem for what it is. Denial runs rampant among drug abusers. Perhaps it is a function of reinforcement: the more we use drugs, the more we want them, and the less willing we are even to entertain the notion of giving them up. The most effective way to avoid that possibility is to keep insisting: "I don't have a drug problem."

Ethan L. used street speed or prescription amphetamines that he got from a "diet doctor," plus sometimes Librium or Placidyl to bring him down. He was a florist, serving a chic upper-income clientele, and ever since he and the drugs had "discovered each other," as he liked to say, he felt that his business had improved. He had more energy, and he felt that his flower arrangements were more original.

Ethan had always had a large circle of friends, most of them unaccustomed to serious drug use. Many were alarmed by Ethan's increasing drug dependency and changing behavior, not to mention the obvious drain on his income. They began to notice too that Ethan's drinking was on the increase. Ethan would be quick to his own defense: cocaine was a far more expensive habit, he'd tell them, and anyway he had his habit well under control. And no, he didn't know what they were talking about, he hardly drank a thing. One by one his friends departed from Ethan's life, tired of the endless denials, and fed up with his increasingly erratic moods and frenzied behavior. To new friends, Ethan would say that he'd give up the pills as soon as he felt that his business was really established. His old friends, he told them, were all out to get him.

Jerry, Ethan's one remaining old friend, tried to reason with him that he'd been in the flower business now for 3½ years—and that his habit was eating up the profits. And loyal Jerry dared to confess that it was becoming harder and harder to deal with Ethan's ups and downs, his nastiness, his paranoia, his intoxicated self-involvement.

Ethan pooh-poohed Jerry's little speech. He had his pill thing under control, he repeated. He could see that Jerry was out to get him too. And if Jerry was such a puritan about taking a couple of pills in this day and age, he could just take off. Which Jerry did.

Only when Ethan began to have difficulty performing sexually did his denial at last begin to crumble. He was forced to take an honest look at his drug taking and was devastated by what everybody else had tried to warn him about all along. And now, typically, he had nobody to turn to.

OTHER SIGNS, SYMPTOMS, AND SIGNALS

Besides defensiveness and denial, clear signs of difficulty with drugs are:

1. The feeling that the drug you are taking is essential to your normal functioning;
2. Needing increased amounts of it;
3. Experiencing a craving for it;
4. The presence of substance abuse in your or your family's history.

The first three signs point toward dependency, possibly addiction. Adding one or more of these to the fourth, the personal or family history, fairly clinches it: you have a drug problem.

Any change in health, mental functioning, or behavior,

especially if it is sudden, can signal toxicity from drugs. Drug treatment specialists look for any of the signs or symptoms on the following lists, though most of them can have other causes. They are indications that something is wrong:

Physical and Mental

- increased or decreased tolerance for alcohol or drugs
- red face, red nose
- bumps and bruises (from falling or bumping into things)
- puffiness of face or extremities (edema)
- sudden vision difficulties
- swollen nasal membranes
- chest and heart problems, including bronchitis, changed heart rhythms, heart failure
- enlarged liver
- frequent infections of any kind, especially pancreatitis
- digestive problems, including diarrhea, cramping, nausea, vomiting blood
- lingering colds and flu-type symptoms
- high blood pressure
- signs of bad nutrition
- tremors
- blackouts
- changes in reflexes
- loss of coordination
- dizziness
- confusion and slow comprehension
- slurred speech
- memory losses
- anxiety or depression
- delirium
- hallucinations
- insomnia or other sleep disturbance
- impotence or inability to achieve orgasm
- craving for sweets or total avoidance of them
- loss of appetite

Behavioral and Social

- increased reliance on drugs
- family problems
- financial difficulties

- frequent change of jobs or loss of employment; lateness or absenteeism
- car accidents
- increased legal problems (resulting from illegal or anti-social behavior)
- suicidal behavior
- violent behavior
- suspiciousness
- unusually passive behavior
- increase in severity of usual neurotic symptoms

TAKING INVENTORY

The indications can be a great deal more subtle than those listed: maybe an otherwise unexplained pervasive tiredness—or sweating too much—or a vague loss of interest in your lover or spouse.

Take an inventory of your drug use/abuse pattern (see the personal drug-use inventory, pp. 68–69) and see how extensively it intrudes into your life. Particularly with a long-standing pattern the effects are likely to be spotted all over your life.

Alice J. had been taking the same drugs, most of them moderately, for years. Her pattern was common—so common that she was hard-pressed, before taking inventory, to see it as a pattern. At 32 she was well launched on a fast-track career as a network newswriter in New York. Once in a while she'd take Librium, which her psychiatrist prescribed at her request. She'd take 5 to 10 milligrams, a small amount, for a few days when the anxiety—usually something to do with work—was at its worst. The stress would subside, and Alice would go for weeks, occasionally months, without requiring a tranquilizer. And rarely, maybe every few months, Alice would take Dalmane or chloral hydrate to break a sleepless spell. And assorted pain killers—codeine worked best—for those miserable headaches that would attack out of nowhere once or twice a year.

She wasn't much of a drinker, maybe a glass or two of wine with dinner when she was out with her boyfriend Ben or with friends. Besides the four or five cups of coffee she drank during the course of the day, the only drug habit Alice felt she had was her marijuana, of which Alice had at least a puff or two practically every night. She found it helped her relax and let go of the tension of the newsroom. And it was nice, very nice, for sex.

At first the only consequence of her drug-use pattern that Alice could identify was the heavy tiredness she felt late evenings and early mornings. Mornings, in fact, were awful for her. She would wake up feeling as if she had had two hours of sleep, and her face would often be unpleasantly puffy, especially around the eyes. She was having difficulty controlling her weight, since as soon as she'd light up the "munchies" would be upon her. Then there were the sudden attacks of coldness and shivering, which could make bad winters almost unendurable. And if she mixed her medications or marijuana with alcohol—tranquilizer morning and afternoon, wine with dinner, marijuana before bed—the drugged feeling would linger uninvited through the next day. That would spell real trouble, because in that condition Alice couldn't think straight, which would make her fast-paced work especially stressful for her. So she'd come home and smoke a "joint" to relax, which would only make matters worse. Those days she and Ben would almost always have a fight.

Most of the time Alice did a fairly good job of keeping her drug taking under control. Her inventory did reveal a larger marijuana habit than she thought she had—she hadn't been aware that she never went a day without it—but it also allowed her to make sure she didn't go beyond already established levels.

All told, Alice's tracing of her drug-use pattern revealed effects throughout her life, but few compared to what they could have been if she had less control over her behavior.

An inventory taken three months later revealed a very different pattern. Her boyfriend Ben had left. She wasn't expecting it and it knocked out her control. First she needed her Librium, more and more of it, to calm down. Then she couldn't sleep; in came the Dalmane and then chloral hydrate, by prescription. The marijuana was lit earlier and earlier; once she smoked a joint in the ladies' room at work. Wine came with lunch and dinner, and Alice felt bad everywhere she turned. She was logy and stoned and confused and began to take days off from work. At home, she'd get stoned and watch soap operas and refuse to think about anything. But the thoughts crept in—some at the insistence of her therapist. She did a drug inventory

Personal Drug-Use Inventory

This list of questions can help you decide whether you are misusing prescription pills or have the potential for misusing them. There are no "good" or "bad" answers to many of them—only honest answers. But if you find yourself silently answering "yes" to more than a few, it may be time to start thinking about ways to reduce your use of drugs.

Are Drugs Affecting You Financially?

- Has spending money on drugs kept you from buying necessities, such as food or clothing, or from paying the rent or mortgage?
- Do you worry about how you'll pay for the pills you use?
- Have you ever borrowed money to buy drugs?

Are Drugs Affecting Your Work?

- Have you ever missed a day's work because of using drugs?
- Have you ever used drugs for "fun" or to "help get through the day" while at work?
- Do your co-workers use drugs and try to get you to join them?
- Have you been worried lately about losing your job because of your use of drugs?

Do Drugs Get You into Trouble?

- Have you ever driven a car while you've been under the influence of drugs and/or alcohol?
- Have you ever had an accident or been given a ticket while you were using drugs and/or alcohol?
- Have you lost a friend or friends because of your use of prescription drugs?
- Do you lie about your drug use? even to your close friends?
- Do you sometimes argue with people about the way you use drugs?

Do You Use Drugs for Nonmedical Reasons?

- Do you take pills to improve your mood?
- Do you use drugs to improve your sexual performance?
- Do you take drugs to help you forget your problems?
- Do you sometimes take a pill before breakfast, perhaps to get the day off to a "good" start?

Do You Miss Drugs When You Stop Using Them?

- When you don't use drugs for a few days, do you feel depressed?
- Do you feel "left out" when you're not using drugs?
- Do you sometimes feel sick—a headache, upset stomach, etc.—when you stop taking pills for a few days or a couple of weeks?

Does Your Use of Drugs Bother You at Times?

- Have you lost interest in sex—even a little—since you've been using drugs?
- Have you ever stopped taking pills, even temporarily, because of an unpleasant physical or mental feeling?
- Have you ever felt sick while taking drugs but kept on taking them anyway?
- Have you ever tried to cut down your drug use?
- Do you sometimes worry that your drug use is out of control?
- Have you ever wondered whether you're addicted to drugs?
- Do you ever feel guilty about taking drugs?
- Do you have trouble waking up or feel like you have a hangover the morning after you use drugs?
- Do you suspect that your use of drugs has increased over the past few months?
- Do you think about drugs at least once a day? more often than that?

Are Drugs Affecting the Way You Think?

- Have you sometimes thought about suicide since you've been using drugs?
- Do you sometimes accept a pill without even asking what it is when a friend offers it to you?
- Are you sometimes unable to remember what happened after you've used drugs?
- Do you have trouble concentrating when you've taken pills?

and got the picture of what she was doing and what it was doing to her. Her self-disgust was enough to shock her controls back into operation.

EVALUATING THE PATTERN AND DECIDING WHAT TO DO

If your pattern leads you to think that you are dependent on drugs, or if it reveals serious consequences in any life area, you have basically two choices:

1. Reestablish control or institute new rules and return to safe use.

2. Stop taking the drug or drugs altogether—a sure test of how dependent or addicted you are. (And if you can't even consider stopping, even for a week or two, that's another sure indication of the extent of the drug's hold over you.)

Addicts and predisposed individuals will have no choice; they will have to go off and stay off in order to avoid further problems. This is best accomplished by entering into a recovery program and living a comfortable life without psychoactive drugs.

STOPPING

The safest way to go off any drug is to taper off slowly so that body and mind will be able to resume natural functioning once the drug has cleared the system. Tapering takes control, however, and with the more reinforcing drugs— like amphetamines or cocaine—it takes an iron constitution to make do with less and less each time. It is easier to stop and avoid further exposure. But with drugs that produce physical dependency, particularly the sedatives (including the benzodiazepine tranquilizers), abruptly stopping—"cold turkey"—may not be safe. It can trigger a severe abstinence (withdrawal) syndrome. To prevent this, seek medical supervision at a hospital or private detoxification program under the guidance of your doctor (see chapter 5).

If you take yourself off drugs, suddenly or gradually, and symptoms of withdrawal begin, take the drug once more and the syndrome will cease. Then seek supervision.

Drugs which promote primarily psychological reliance are safely stopped cold turkey. Be prepared to endure a few days or weeks of feeling depressed or sleepless or angry. This will subside. But you still may wish to be under supervision; if so, see chapter 5.

CONTROLLING DRUG USE

It is possible to change a drug use or abuse pattern that has not developed into compulsive use or addiction by changing or manipulating any of the variables mentioned in the first two chapters. Any change will alter the pattern in some way.

Identify the most significant factors (using the self-monitoring questionnaire) and work with them first. Since drug dependency and toxicity are always (except for the susceptible ten-percenters) dose- and frequency-related, many of the problems will diminish or disappear, temptation included, when the dose is cut or when the doctor's instructions are more closely followed. One woman discovered to her surprise that when she smoked unusually potent marijuana she would experience a powerful craving for other drugs as well. But when she smoked a weaker strain of marijuana, she had no further problems.

Tolerance can be manipulated by taking "therapeutic breaks" every now and then. No matter which drug is being taken, or who's prescribing it, psychoactive pill taking should be stopped (tapered off slowly) for at least a few weeks every two to three months, depending on the medication, to let the accumulated effects of tolerance and dependency subside.

State-dependent learning can be similarly skirted by alternating the pattern of use so that an activity and the drug are never consistently paired. With those drugs that enhance sexual performance or experience, keep in practice without the drug too. Artists and performers, whose horns blow so sweetly with just a couple of pills, should make sure often to naturally wet their whistles to avoid the state-dependence trap.

Some of the worst toxic effects of drug use can be eliminated by altering the mixture of drugs. Sometimes just doing without alcohol is enough. Or keep the alcohol and eliminate the drugs.

Controlling drug use almost always means grappling with temptation. *Availability* is often the key factor. If the drug is right there you'll take it; but would you walk a mile for it? If you don't carry your pills with you, you won't have them around all the time to take.

Changing the *setting* may work. It did for John R., who kept getting in car accidents when he was stoned on Percodan, a potent pain killer, prescribed for a back injury years back when he played professional football. Actually, the state changed the setting for John by removing his driver's license. After six months of no wheels, John learned it was possible to get around by bus and taxi. When his license was reinstated, he was able to stay out of harm's way by driving less. It was either that or go off the drug, and that much John still wasn't prepared to do.

In times of *stress*, instead of increasing your drug use, be vigilant about using other, natural stress reduction techniques (see "Appropriate Use of Psychoactive Drugs," p. 77).

Or the critical variables may be *social*. Groups of friends or relationships identified with drug taking may have to be left behind. Margaret S. left her boyfriend—she knew that was the only way she was ever going to lighten her narcotics load. He wanted her to shoot up and do pills with him, didn't want her to stop, became abusive when she brought the subject up. She once even prostituted herself with his blessing when they couldn't come up with enough money for drugs. Leaving him was rough, but once she did she found she had far less of a problem getting off drugs than she had ever imagined. She did seek help at a free clinic, joined a rap group of other users, and buttressed her support system.

CONTROLLING DRUG HUNGER

As those who diet know, hunger is very difficult to manipulate or control, and the more you indulge yourself in food, the harder it is to feel satiated with less. The same is true with drugs. Whether for food or for drugs, hunger is psychobiological—no doubt influenced by neurotransmitters, although the mechanisms are not clear.

Drug hunger and compulsive use go hand in hand: hunger is the urge and compulsive use the behavior that develops to satisfy it. Eventually, uncontrolled feeding of drug hunger will lead to all the worst consequences of drug abuse, including addiction. Drug hunger is a sign and a result of addictive disease.

The only guaranteed way to deal with drug hunger is to keep it from arising. Never count on your ability to wrestle with a drug craving each time it happens. Repeated self-monitoring of dosage, frequency, and effects can help you head off the problem at the pass. By keeping track of the changes in your pattern of drug taking, it serves a purpose similar to that of a scale for a potential food abuser.

DRUGS IN THE FAMILY

Through lost jobs, changes in expression of affection, aggression, and emotion, the whole family suffers the consequences of a member's drug abuse. The family may also be the primary "variable" out of which drug abuse springs. Patterns of drug abuse are passed from generation to generation, via genetic factors, learning, or both.

Mike B.'s mother's drug abuse pattern was so subtle he never put two and two together when he lived at home. She rarely drank—only at parties—and the pills she took were all prescribed. But her medicine cabinet and one drawer in the kitchen were always loaded with pill bottles. When Miltown, the first of the modern tranquilizers, came out in the 1950s, Mike's mom was asking her doctor for it in no time. She was a tense, driven woman, and her doctors saw no reason why they should not try to help her relax and get to sleep. She drank a lot of coffee, smoked, and frequently dieted, taking a variety of amphetamines.

Mike's father didn't use any drugs or drink. His wife wished he would—she thought it would calm his temper and relax him. Brutal fights between his parents were common when Mike was young. Once, when he was eight, Mike and his four-year-old sister Linda cowered unseen, crying, while his father bloodied his mother's nose. During a sudden silence some minutes later, the mother, hearing how upset her children were, rushed to telephone their pediatrician to prescribe a sedative for them. He complied, ordering phenobarbital. Some years later, when Linda's first big crush broke her heart, more of the sedative was prescribed to calm her. This was about the time too, Mike remembered, when Linda began to be aware of her

chubbiness; the pediatrician, at the mother's behest, prescribed Dexamyl.

Mike took pills himself only when he had colds or a sore
throat. He didn't even like aspirin. And he didn't seem to
suffer the emotional upsets that Linda did. Mike went away
to college when Linda was 14. Through the years, living in
different cities, he and Linda grew apart.

Her apparent suicide years later forced him to come to
terms with his family's pattern of pill taking. Linda was 30
and her marriage had broken up days before. She had
overdosed on what doctors estimated to be literally hundreds of barbiturates and tranquilizers, all from legal prescriptions filled and kept over a period of years. His first
shocked question was: What was she doing with so many
pills? The tragic pattern soon became clear. Pills for escape
from pain, anger, tension, frustration, hurt—Mike's mother
had started Linda on a pill-taking pattern that ended in her
permanent escape from everything.

The Family's Involvement

As in Mike's family, drug abuse, particularly of prescription drugs, may not be seen for what it is. And denial can
operate on the group level too.

Many families deny that there is any problem with drugs.
Others may recognize that one member has a drug problem but will deny that the family as a whole is troubled.
Family therapists believe that certain families unconsciously
have a vested interest in keeping the drug-abusing member on drugs. They use the drug abuser as a scapegoat,
pointing to him or her as "the problem" or as the one
responsible for all their problems. If the drug abuser man-
ages nonetheless to break free of drugs, another member
of the family may all of a sudden develop a drug problem!
Because of this, and because drug abuse is a terrible drain
on a family's emotional and financial resources, family
therapy is often recommended. Al-Anon, a self-help organization for relatives and friends of alcoholics and other
substance abusers, can help you deal with the consequences
of another person's drug abuse, and can help you identify
how you contribute—or how you don't—to the problem.
Information on Al-Anon and family therapy, along with
other avenues of help, is provided in chapter 5.

Recognizing the Signs

You may have a strong suspicion but not know how to tell if drugs have crept into your family. And with drugs so available to children, it is hard to know whether a substance is causing them to act as they do or if adolescence is the culprit.

The signs and symptoms listed on pages 64–66 are useful but not conclusive. Look for any sudden, drastic change in health or behavior—with a child, a sudden unexplained drop in grades; with an adult, a sudden need for large sums of money, or unusual emotional displays. Frequent brief disappearances from the room, with a return in a different mood, may be telling. Sudden change in attention to dress and grooming, new eating habits, excuse making, lying, can all be signs of other difficulties, but if you think drugs could be involved: ask.

Confrontation

Reactions will vary from indignation to outrage to honest denial to honest confession—often depending on how the question is delivered. Be supportive and nonthreatening. Say what you have noticed—the moodiness, the slipped grades, the absenteeism, the euphoria, the drowsiness. Offer a willingness to listen and to help in finding a solution. Try not to judge the behavior but to see it as a problem. Address the problem or factors that may contribute to the drug abuse—a child's poor opinion of himself or herself, loneliness, boredom, or simply unchecked availability. If the child's problem is a reflection of a parent's own drug difficulty, or symptomatic of a breakdown in the family, be prepared to face your own involvement and to consider seeking help for the entire family. Family therapy is equally appropriate when the adult or adults are the abusers.

The child's school may be able to provide help or information. Educators are often grateful to be able to work with parents on behalf of the children. Contact the teacher or administrator who is in the best position to know about your child's behavior and to work with him or her. Usually it is *not* advisable to contact an employer, but if there is an Employee Assistance Program where your family drug abuser works, recommend that he or she seek help. These programs are confidential and often good sources for referral to drug programs in the community.

Intervention

When denial is stubborn and strong, some drug counselors and self-help organizations recommend a technique called "intervention." The point is not to wring a confession but to force the drug abuser to face up to the problem and do something about it.

For an intervention, gather together as many people as possible who truly *care* about the person—close people from work, friends, the family doctor, family members. Have them present to deliver carefully documented, undeniable evidence of drug abuse or drug abuse behavior. If you can find the drugs themselves, or paraphernalia, bring them. Testify to days of work missed and sloppiness of projects, productivity, or performance. Have the children remind Daddy of his "talking funny" and all his broken promises. Be blunt, supply all the details, but deliver them as an act of kindness. Everyone is there to help—all you hold against the person is the drug.

If your drug abuser insists, despite all the gory details from his boss and his sister, his wife, his mother, his best friend, and his two children, that he doesn't have a problem, challenge him: "Howie, if that drug is no problem to you as you say, prove it—go off the stuff." But if he (or she) begins to rationalize the drug use ("I only do that because . . ."), recognize that he is beginning to admit to a problem.

Don't be afraid to intervene in less formal ways. Call the doctor who is prescribing the pills you believe are being abused; say there is a possible problem and suggest strongly that he or she check it out when the patient next comes by or calls for a prescription. (The doctor's responsibilities, ethical and legal, are covered in chapter 6.) Your responsibilities toward someone you love who goes off the deep end with drugs go as far as you are willing to take them. But only the drug abuser can control the behavior. The most you can do is provide help, love, support, and self-scrutiny, and to agree to work together toward change.

APPROPRIATE USE OF PSYCHOACTIVE DRUGS

Trying to define what is appropriate use of drugs or a drug in particular gets us back to where we started: what is "right" often depends on society's attitude toward intoxicants and intoxicated people.

In terms of safety, however, for most people appropriate use of psychoactive substances means keeping it to a short course at the lowest effective dosage. For the addicted or addiction-prone, use may be appropriate only in a medical emergency. Short of that, in situations where another person might safely (although not necessarily legally) take a drug—pain killers and tranquilizers for a tennis injury, Valium or a stimulant during exam week—an addict or predisposed individual will have to turn to natural, nondrug alternatives. Meditation, acupuncture, massage, heat therapy, relaxation techniques, hypnosis, biofeedback, exercise programs—whatever works to relax, calm, energize, or lessen pain naturally or mechanically is recommended. (Some of these techniques, including acupuncture, are also used in detoxification and to treat continuing drug hunger; see chapter 5.)

Natural ways of coping may also come in handy for the nonaddicted majority who wish to break a long-term pattern of using pills to cope with the mundane miseries of life—big presentation, important date, family blowup, slump in the stock market. Drug treatment specialists as well as drug companies have begun to recommend to doctors that they not prescribe for these "situational anxiety" states, but only for severe anxiety or physical states that truly interfere with functioning. Valium may be appropriate for the first few days of deep emotional shock following the sudden death of a loved one. But it should soon be discontinued and the natural coping mechanisms, say therapists, encouraged to operate; for the actual, miserable experience of pain and anxiety is essential to survival. Writes British medical researcher John Marks in a text on the benzodiazepines written for physicians: "Anxiety is a normal emotion and serves in nature as a valuable function inducing beneficial adaptive change. The intervention of treatment merely to suppress anxiety will prevent or retard the appropriate adaptation and may do more harm than good." Medication to reduce anxiety, he states, will have greatest benefit when ability to function and perform begins to be impaired. This point varies for everybody, but prescribing antianxiety pills before that point is reached can lead to stunting of a person's survival mechanisms. *Given a pill at every emotional crisis, who can learn how to endure, grow from, and transcend the pain of life?*

This is the most far-reaching consequence of children's drug use. If Stevie starts taking pills in junior high when life is beginning to reveal its stresses, he'll never build his coping muscles for when he truly needs them. Drugs, say counselors and therapists, lure kids into thinking that life is supposed to provide quick relief and easy answers. They never learn to wait the few weeks it might take for the worst of a heartbreak or disappointment to subside. Drugs do not correct anything. All they do is alter the reaction.

"The causal therapy for the patient mentally disturbed by stress is the removal of the stress, not the suppression of its manifestations." Dr. Marks admonishes his colleagues.

Going off drugs can itself be highly stressful. To remove *this* stress may require outside assistance. How to get assistance is the subject of the next chapter.

5
Getting Help

The number of services available for drug abusers and addicts is huge and ever-growing. There are hospital detoxification units, residential medical/psychological drug treatment centers, therapeutic communities, outpatient clinics and counseling centers, community outreach programs, self-help support groups, crisis hotlines, and individual doctors and therapists.

Approaches to detoxification and treatment are varied. Some insist on total abstinence even during the withdrawal period ("cold turkey") and disdain use of any medications, aspirin included. Others (specifically, methadone maintenance clinics) substitute one, more controlled addiction for the original one. Still others are satisfied if they change an individual's drug use pattern into a less destructive one.

SOURCES OF INFORMATION

All 50 states have substance abuse agencies which coordinate information on available drug treatment facilities and programs. The best sources of information on local options are the city, county, or community coordinators of these agencies. (See pp. 87–91 for the name and address of the appropriate agency for each state.) If there is no listing for that agency in your local telephone directory, write or phone the state office for the local coordinator to contact. *These coordinators are not connected with law enforcement.* They are there to direct you to the appropriate resources and are not interested in reporting you for drug use.

Your doctor may know about these programs and may be able to match you to one best suited to your problem and your personality.

Hospitals, social service departments, community mental health associations, professional medical and psychological associations, school guidance departments, Employee Assistance Programs, and religious institutions are other good sources of information. For "alternative" treatment and referrals methods, try the American Holistic Medical Association (6932 Little River Turnpike, Annandale, VA 22003; [703] 642-5880). Crisis hotlines (call directory assistance) are often good referral sources.

WHAT DO YOU WANT OR NEED?

In general, there are two aspects of drug treatment: detoxification and counseling/rehabilitation. Programs or approaches which do not aid with adjustment to a drug-free life-style are the least effective in keeping clients off drugs in the long run. The hardest part of the process is *staying* off.

Because there are so many approaches and programs, it is best to begin thinking now about what you are willing to do to conquer your drug problem and what you wish to accomplish.

- Do you want to end your drug use or only to modify it?
- Are you willing to give up all drugs or only the drug with which you are having the problem?
- Are you willing to change your life-style, even give up your friends?
- Are you willing to move into a hospital or facility?
- Do you want drug detoxification, counseling, or drug detoxification with counseling?
- How are you at following orders?
- How motivated are you to change?
- Have you tried to stop or to change your drug habits in the past? If so, which approaches or treatment (or aspects of them) seemed to work best for you, and which failed?

Be as realistic as possible about who you are, what you want, and what you are likely to accomplish, in order to choose the approach that is best tailored to your needs and goals. If you are a loner and do not care to affiliate with groups, there is little point in joining a therapeutic community which will insist on your total commitment to the "family." If your goal is only to cut back, you are wasting your time at Alcoholics Anonymous.

DETOXIFICATION AND WITHDRAWAL
METHODS AND RESOURCES

The procedures used to withdraw a physically dependent user from a drug are called detoxification. Methods used vary depending on the doctor or program and on the drug. In "cold turkey" you stop taking the drug and endure the resulting abstinence syndrome until it is over. Some programs will not prescribe medications to ease or aid the withdrawal; some will. Medically based programs will, of course, assist in easing the symptoms and making the experience as comfortable and as safe as possible.

In medical detoxification of sedative-hypnotics which produce physical dependence and have a substantial risk of withdrawal seizures, administered by physicians, the principle is to slowly detoxify you from the drug of abuse by administering steadily decreasing doses of the drug, or by substituting another drug and then steadily decreasing its dosage. The substituted drug is one to which you are cross-tolerant but which is less toxic and has a lower addiction potential than the one you have been taking. (Cross-tolerant substances will meet the same dependency need of body cells and therefore forestall withdrawal; the term "cross-dependence" is sometimes used in this context.) Phenobarbital, a slower-acting, low-potency barbiturate, is often used for withdrawal from alcohol, minor tranquilizers, and sedatives. The substituted drug is first administered just to the point of intoxication, then steadily lessened.

Methadone, a drug cross-tolerant to narcotics, is often used to detoxify heroin addicts and as a substitute drug. Methadone, however, is as toxic as heroin and higher in addiction potential. The methadone is administered to stabilize withdrawal, not to promote euphoria (although clients often report that it makes them high). The patient takes 10–40 mg. of methadone in a gradual reduction program for 21 days and then is discontinued, thus avoiding methadone addiction.

During detoxification, medication may also be provided for anxiety and depression. In treating alcoholics and sedative addicts this is controversial, however, in light of cross-addictive possibilities.

Detoxification or withdrawal procedures are listed for each drug in section II. If you are dependent on sedatives (tranquilizers included), you should usually be hospitalized for the detoxification period. If a residential program has 24-hour on-site medical supervision, it is safe to withdraw from sedatives on the premises. Hospital detoxification is recommended if you are pregnant or at risk of exacerbating a medical or psychiatric condition.

Inpatient detoxification generally lasts three to six weeks. Some medical insurance policies offer coverage for this type of treatment.

Outpatient facilities, such as free clinics or other drug treatment facilities, can provide sufficient, and cheaper, supervision of withdrawal from all other drugs.

Outpatient treatment is sufficient for drugs that promote primarily psychological dependency, but inpatient programs may be desirable. Just because the withdrawal is not physical doesn't mean it is comfortable or easy. Stimulant users with long-standing, high-dose habits may have to contend with serious depression during withdrawal. Antidepressants may be required. If you feel the least bit suicidal, supervision is essential.

Private physicians, sometimes those specializing in toxicology, may also provide detoxification or treatment. These specialists are often consulted by long-time users who have no intention of quitting; they want to reduce their tolerance to the drug and return to a more effective, less harmful, lower dose. Your local medical association may be a source of information about toxicologists or other specialists who treat drug-using patients in this way. (Word-of-mouth is probably better.) Other detoxification resources may be used to achieve this goal, but make sure first that their philosophy does not preclude it.

THERAPEUTIC COMMUNITIES

These are nonmedical residential self-help programs based originally on the Synanon model, the California therapeutic community founded by Charles Dederich, a recovered alcoholic, in the late 1950s. Dederich and his followers demonstrated that it was possible for addicts to remain drug free and to reenter the workaday world. These days, Synanon's goals (and those of some other communities patterned after it) have changed significantly. Residents are encouraged to remain within the community rather than to rejoin society at large. Some such communities may be cultish and demand unflagging devotion to a charismatic leader. Many therapeutic communities demand strict adherence to their rules and regulations; this disciplined commitment is often the basis for their success.

Therapeutic communities generally require absolute abstinence from all drugs. Some insist on cold turkey withdrawal. Residence lasts up to two years, during which all activities are centered around the community and acquiring new drug-free habits. Group therapy is often the principal treatment technique. Newcomers have the lowest status and must prove themselves worthy of privileges. The atmosphere can be that of a loving family with strong, positive values. In this way a good therapeutic community can accomplish a total change in life-style and commitment to a new life. Therapeutic communities exclusively for medical professionals can be highly effective in helping doctors and nurses change their drug habits while remaining within the medical "family."

Because therapeutic communities can vary so widely, in cost as well as in philosophy and treatment methods, it is essential to inspect them closely. Find out exactly how the community is run, who is on the board of directors (do they represent leading human services representatives from the community?), whether there are medical services and/or on-call medical consultants. Does the community have a leader or leadership? What are the qualifications of staff members? Ask them to specify their values, follow-up success rates, exact approach, and goals, and their expectations from new members.

OUTPATIENT CLINICS

Called anything from free clinics to community clinics to drug-free clinics, these offer a wide range of walk-in treatment services, often free of charge. These clinics are good resources for the withdrawal period of opiates, amphetamines, and cocaine. Some provide medication for symptomatic relief during withdrawal; the "drug-free" ones will refer you to other resources. Based on the model of the San Francisco Haight-Ashbury Free Clinic, which was the first (1967), free clinics often provide a wide range of medical, psychotherapeutic, and self-help services for drug abusers and families of drug abusers in a "nonestablishment" atmosphere. Some also provide or recommend "alternative" treatments, such as acupuncture.

The overall trend in outpatient care is to provide treatment tailored to the specific needs of the client, as ascertained in the intake interview. These facilities can be the best resources for crucial ongoing support.

METHADONE MAINTENANCE CLINICS

Replacing heroin addiction with addiction to methadone, these clinics are best seen as a last resort when all attempts to stop fail. Being addicted to a legal substance rather than an illegal one is the only way some addicts can rehabilitate themselves and resume productive lives. In Great Britain, where addicts may receive heroin from government-controlled clinics, their addiction need not force them into criminal activity and constant anxiety over whether they will be able to obtain a supply. In the U.S. the only legal narcotics addiction is methadone maintenance. It is used principally because it is a drug which blocks heroin from the opiate receptors and is effective in an oral dose form. It suppresses the addict's narcotics hunger, and heroin has no effect while taking methadone in a replacement/maintenance program. Most methadone maintenance clinics offer some counseling, and all require frequent urine tests to monitor drug levels in the system. Some reports quote a 40 to 60 percent success rate in keeping addicts from returning to heroin. The clinics are willing to help an addict detoxify from methadone when he or she is ready; but this is rarely accomplished. Methadone, it has been discovered, is much more difficult to withdraw from than heroin and the process can take many months. (Methadone is also a much desired street drug, considered "better" than heroin.)

ALTERNATIVE APPROACHES

"The fact remains," says the AMA's *Drug Abuse, A Guide for the Primary Care Physician*, "that no single treatment method yet devised has solved, or promises to solve, all of the complex problems involved in drug abuse. There still is confusion and controversy about the nature of drug dependence and how society should deal with it. Ideally, a vari-

ety of methods and approaches should be available to help
the multitude of people who abuse drugs today."

Indeed, the methods are multiplying and some approaches
previously considered "far out" are taking their place along-
side standard treatment, detoxification, and rehabilitation
techniques in drug clinics. These include hypnosis, acupuncture, biofeedback, and behavior modification techniques
for conditioning to new habits and dealing with drug craving.
An innovative method involving mild electric currents delivered through electrodes taped behind the ears is claimed
to have helped such rock stars as Keith Richards, Eric
Clapton, and Peter Townshend of The Who to successfully
end their long-term drug addictions. Devised by Dr. Margaret Patterson, a Scottish surgeon now living in southern
California, the method is called NeuroElectric Therapy (NET)
and adherents claim it is particularly successful in helping
end drug craving. Acupuncture treatment, used by such
programs as the Haight-Ashbury Free Medical Clinic, has
similar results to the NeuroElectric Therapy. It's thought
that a similar biochemical reaction occurs. Like all detoxification procedures, this produces best results when combined with psychotherapy or counseling and retraining for
a new life-style.

SELF-HELP

No one knows more about getting off and staying off
drugs than someone who has successfully done both. And
no one is better equipped than a recovering addict or
alcoholic to understand the struggle. Self-help approaches,
based on pooled experience and mutual support, are increasingly widespread.

The grandfather of this method is Alcoholics Anonymous (which now deals with other addictions too, since
alcoholics are frequently involved with other substances).
AA is a self-help organization run entirely by recovered or
recovering alcoholics. Its network is worldwide and reaches
into almost every community in the U.S. AA requires total
abstinence and has a spiritual orientation (no particular
religion is espoused). It provides a specific program to
follow as well as the critical variable that most addicts
require to get off and stay off the substance: each other.
AA provides round-the-clock assistance. If there is no list-

ing in your telephone book, write Alcoholics Anonymous, P.O. Box 459, Grand Central Station, New York, NY 10017. Organizations related to AA include Narcotics Anonymous (NA) and Pills Anonymous; and, for families and loved ones of abusers: Al-Anon, Alateen, Children of Alcoholics (for adults whose parents were or are alcoholics), and Pil-Anon. AA is a good source of information about detoxification and medical problems associated with substance abuse.

Recognizing the efficacy of self-help and mutual aid, drug treatment centers and clinics increasingly sponsor support and identification groups. It is also possible to start your own group and to work with your own friends in getting off and staying off. For information on how to form and run your own group, contact the National Self-Help Clearinghouse (33 W. 42 St., Rm. 1206-A, New York, NY 10036); or the Self-Help Center (1600 Dodge Ave., Suite S-122, Evanston, IL 60201).

The Clearinghouse will also help you locate existing self-help groups. Send a stamped self-addressed envelope and state the nature of your problem. They will reply with information about national organizations to contact, which in turn will supply addresses of local resources.

The Self-Help Center provides a similar service, but is best equipped for the Chicago metropolitan area.

PSYCHOTHERAPY

Knowledge among psychotherapists about drug abuse varies. If you consult a therapist specifically for a drug problem, it is best to obtain a referral from a drug treatment clinic or organization; that way you'll ensure that the therapist will be knowledgeable and sympathetic to your problem. Psychotherapy is often useful as an adjunct to other treatments to help you work out the problems that contributed to your drug abuse and those which have resulted from it. Family therapy is lately seen as advantageous in producing lasting change, for the family is the environment from which the drug abuser comes and often must return.

ALABAMA
Div. of Alcoholism and Drug
  Abuse
Dept. of Mental Health
135 S. Union St.
Montgomery 36130
(205) 265-2301

ALASKA
Office of Alcoholism and Drug
  Abuse
Pouch H-05-F
Juneau 99811
(907) 586-6201

ARIZONA
Drug Abuse Section
Dept. of Health Services
2500 East Van Buren
Phoenix 85008
(602) 255-1239

ARKANSAS
Office on Alcohol and Drug
  Abuse Prevention
Suite 310
1515 W. 7th St.
Little Rock 72202
(501) 371-2604

CALIFORNIA
Dept. of Alcohol and Drug Abuse
111 Capital Mall
Sacramento 95814
(916) 322-2974

COLORADO
Alcoholism and Drug Abuse Div.
Dept. of Health
4210 E. 11th Ave.
Denver 80220
(303) 320-8333

CONNECTICUT
Alcohol and Drug Abuse
  Commission
999 Asylum Ave.
Hartford 06105
(203) 566-4145

DELAWARE
Bureau of Alcoholism and Drug
  Abuse
1901 N. DuPont Hwy.
Newcastle 19720
(302) 421-6101

DISTRICT OF COLUMBIA
Department of Human Services
Office of Health Planning and
  Development
601 Indiana Ave., N.W.
Washington, D.C. 20004
(202) 724-5641

FLORIDA
Drug Abuse Program
1317 Winewood Blvd.
Tallahassee 32301
(904) 488-0900

GEORGIA
Alcoholism and Drug Abuse
  Section
Div. of Mental Health & Mental
  Retardation
878 Peachtree St.
Atlanta 30309
(404) 894-4204

HAWAII
Alcohol and Drug Abuse Branch
1270 Queen Emma St.
Honolulu 96813
(808) 548-7655

IDAHO
Bureau of Substance Abuse
450 W. State
Boise 83720
(208) 334-4368

ILLINOIS
Dangerous Drugs Commission
300 N. State St.
Chicago 60610
(312) 822-9860

INDIANA
Div. of Addiction Services
Dept. of Mental Health
429 N. Pennsylvania
Indianapolis 46204
(317) 232-7816

IOWA
Dept. of Substance Abuse
505 Fifth Ave.
Des Moines 50319
(515) 281-3641

KANSAS
Dept. of Social Rehabilitation
Services
Alcohol & Drug Abuse Services
2700 W. Sixth St.
Topeka 66606
(913) 296-3925

KENTUCKY
Cabinet for Human Resources
Dept. of Substance Abuse
275 E. Main St.
Frankfort 40621
(502) 564-2880

LOUISIANA
Office of Mental Health and Sub-
stance Abuse
P.O. Box 4049
Baton Rouge 70821
(504) 342-2575

MAINE
Office of Alcoholism and Drug
Abuse Prevention
32 Winthrop St.
Augusta 04330
(207) 289-2781

MARYLAND
State Drug Abuse Administration
201 W. Preston St.
Baltimore 21201
(301) 282-7404

MASSACHUSETTS
Div. of Drug Rehabilitation
160 N. Washington St.
Boston 02114
(617) 727-8614

MICHIGAN
Office of Substance Abuse Ser
vices
Dept. of Public Health
3500 N. Logan St.
Lansing 48909
(517) 373-8600

MINNESOTA
Chemical Dependency Program
Div.
Dept. of Public Welfare
568 Cedar
St. Paul 55155
(612) 296-4610

MISSISSIPPI
Div. of Alcohol & Drug Abuse
Dept. of Mental Health
1102 Robert E. Lee State Office
Bldg.
Jackson 39201
(601) 359-1297

MISSOURI
Div. of Alcoholism and Drug Abuse
Dept. of Mental Health
2002 Missouri Blvd.
P.O. Box 687
Jefferson City 65102
(314) 751-4942

MONTANA
Alcohol & Drug Abuse Div.
Dept. of Institutions
1539 11th Ave.
Helena 59620
(406) 449-2827

NEBRASKA
Div. on Alcoholism and Drug Abuse
P.O. Box 94728
Lincoln 68509
(402) 471-2851

NEVADA
Bureau of Alcohol & Drug Abuse
505 E. King St.
Carson City 89710
(702) 885-4790

NEW HAMPSHIRE
State Alcohol & Drug Abuse Program
Hazen Drive
Concord 03301
(603) 271-4630

NEW JERSEY
Div. of Narcotic & Drug Abuse Control
129 E. Hanover St.
Trenton 08625
(609) 292-5760

NEW MEXICO
Substance Abuse Bureau
Behavioral Services Div.
Crown Building
P.O. Box 968
Santa Fe 87503
(505) 984-0020

NEW YORK
Div. of Substance Abuse Services
Executive Park S.
Box 8200
Albany 12203
(518) 457-7629

NORTH CAROLINA
Alcohol and Drug Abuse Section
Dept. of Human Resources
325 N. Salisbury St.
Raleigh 27611
(919) 733-4670

NORTH DAKOTA
Div. of Alcoholism & Drug Abuse
Dept. of Human Services
State Capitol
Bismarck 58505
(701) 224-2767

OHIO
Bureau of Drug Abuse
65 S. Front St.
Columbus 43215
(614) 466-9023

OKLAHOMA
Drug Abuse Services
Dept. of Mental Health
P.O. Box 53277, Capitol Station
Oklahoma City 73152
(405) 521-0044

OREGON
Dept. of Human Resources
Mental Health Div.
Office of Programs for Alcohol & Drug Problems
2575 Bittern St., N.E.
Salem 97310
(503) 378-2163

PENNSYLVANIA
Office of Drug and Alcohol Programs
Dept. of Health
Health and Welfare Building
Harrisburg 17108
(717) 787-9857

RHODE ISLAND
Div. of Substance Abuse
Rhode Island Medical Center
Substance Administration
   Building
Cranston 02920
(401) 464-2091

SOUTH CAROLINA
Commission on Alcohol & Drug
   Abuse
3700 Forest Dr.
Columbia 29204
(803) 758-2521

SOUTH DAKOTA
Div. of Alcohol and Drug Abuse
523 E. Capitol
Joe Foss Bldg.
Pierre 57501
(605) 773-3123

TENNESSEE
Alcohol & Drug Abuse Services
505 Deaderick St.
James K. Polk Bldg.
Nashville 37219
(615) 741-1921

TEXAS
Drug Abuse Prevention Div.
Dept. of Community Affairs
P.O. Box 13166
Austin 78711
(512) 443-4100

UTAH
Div. of Alcoholism & Drugs
P.O. Box 2500
Salt Lake City 84110
(801) 533-6532

VERMONT
Alcohol & Drug Abuse Div.
Dept. of Social & Rehabilitation
   Services
103 S. Main St.
Waterbury 05676
(802) 241-2175

VIRGINIA
Div. of Substance Abuse
Dept. of Mental Rehabilitation
   & Retardation
109 Governor St.
P.O. Box 1797
Richmond 23214
(804) 786-5313

WASHINGTON
Bureau of Alcohol & Substance
   Abuse
Dept. of Social & Health Services
   Office Bldg.
Mail Stop OB-44W
Olympia 98504
(206) 753-3073

WEST VIRGINIA
Div. of Alcohol and Drug Abuse
State Capitol
1800 Kanawha Blvd. E
Charleston 25305
(304) 348-3616

WISCONSIN
Office of Alcohol & Other Drug
   Abuse
P.O. Box 7851
One W. Wilson St.
Madison 53707
(608) 266-2717

WYOMING
Div. of Community Programs
Substance Abuse Programs
Hathaway Bldg.
Cheyenne 82002
(307) 777-7118

PUERTO RICO
Dept. of Addiction Control Ser-
   vices
Alcohol and Drug Abuse
   Programs
Box B-Y, Rio Piedras Station
Rio Piedras 00928
(809) 763-5014

AMERICAN SAMOA
LBJ Tropical Medical Center
Dept. of Mental Health Clinic
Pago Pago 96799

GUAM
Mental Health & Substance
  Abuse Agency
P.O. Box 20999
Guam 96921

VIRGIN ISLANDS
Div. of Mental Health, Alcohol-
  ism & Drug Dependency
  Services
P.O. Box 7329
St. Thomas 00801
(809) 774-7265

TRUST TERRITORIES
Director of Health Services
Office of the High Commissioner
Saipan 96950

Source: *National Directory of Drug Abuse and Alcoholism Treat-
ment Programs.* (U.S. Department of Health and Human Services;
National Institute on Drug Abuse and National Institute on Alcohol
Abuse and Alcoholism)

6
The Doctor's Responsibilities— and Your Own

A physician is bound by more than medical training when prescribing pills to a patient. Certainly a doctor is obligated to try to diagnose a patient's condition and, after diagnosis, to treat it—through medication, surgery, or other means—as effectively as possible.

Many of a physician's responsibilities are spelled out by laws and professional regulations which require the doctor to follow certain guidelines when prescribing medications, or risk losing his license or being dragged into court on malpractice charges.

Most pills are prescribed in accordance with accepted medical standards. They represent the appropriate treatment for a known or suspected medical condition. Many other prescriptions are of questionable wisdom, however. Statistics show that thousands of doctors routinely prescribe certain drugs—especially tranquilizers—for just about every patient who claims to have trouble getting to sleep. Doctors also often prescribe pills that are unsuitable for the condition being treated; such prescriptions may amount to experimental usage, with the patient unaware he has been used as a guinea pig.

A doctor sometimes prescribes a medication that is hazardous to the patient because of allergy to it, or some physical condition which should rule it out.

From time to time drugs are even prescribed by doctors who haven't bothered to check the patient's health record or prior experience with medications. The results can be tragic.

In a recent case a Connecticut woman was given the pain killer ibuprofen (Motrin), and suffered a severe allergic reaction resulting in her death a few hours later. Medical references warn that the drug should not be used by anyone sensitive to aspirin, and the woman's medical records plainly noted she was allergic to aspirin. After her death her husband and children accepted an out-of-court settlement of $680,000 from her doctor's insurance company, although the family had not filed a malpractice suit.

Laws and regulations require the doctor to practice medicine at least as well as an average physician in the same or a similar community. If the doctor who prescribed your tranquilizer is a general practitioner, the choice of drug—and the decision to use a medication at all—should result from at least the level of expertise possessed by other general practitioners in the same area or a similar area.

The tranquilizer doesn't have to be the *best* medication available. If the majority of physicians in your community prescribe it for most patients complaining of mild insomnia, and if it is suggested by the manufacturer—and approved by the government—as a possible treatment for insomnia, then the prescription most likely meets the "average physician" standard.

A 50-year-old New York man suffering from depression recently discovered how the wrong pills can be prescribed by large numbers of doctors with very little liability. Martin B. consulted a psychiatrist about his depression and was given a four-week series of electroshock treatments, without success. Then the psychiatrist prescribed the antipsychotic drug fluphenazine hydrochloride (Prolixin), which Martin B. took faithfully for two years while visiting the psychiatrist every month. Eventually the patient realized the drug was doing him no good and stopped taking it. He also stopped seeing the psychiatrist.

A few weeks later Martin B.'s wife noticed him sticking out his tongue frequently, smacking his lips, and making chewing motions. He seemed unaware of this. His condition was eventually diagnosed as tardive dyskinesia, an occasional adverse reaction to fluphenazine hydrochloride and other antipsychotic drugs. There is no known cure.

Only then did Martin B. learn that the drug he had been given is not considered the best medication for depression, and that many other drugs should have been tried first. Yet hundreds of physicians and psychiatrists prescribe antipsychotic drugs for conditions just like his. Because the drug has *some* potential for helping depressed patients, and because it is commonly used by the medical community, there was no legal recourse against the psychiatrist for prescribing it.

Unfortunately, questions about the wisdom of prescriptions seldom arise until after the pills have proven to be harmful, or even deadly. Even then, physicians with poor pill-prescribing practices seldom face criminal charges. They are occasionally sued for medical malpractice and even less often are investigated by their medical colleagues— who may, in the most serious cases, suspend the errant doctor's license.

You too have certain duties if you want to avoid being harmed by improper pill prescribing. First, tell the doctor everything about yourself. Reveal the extent of your drug or alcohol use, as well as your family's history with drugs and alcohol. Your medical history is strictly confidential; physicians have been successfully sued for revealing details of their patients' medical conditions to people not directly involved in treatment, such as nurses or X-ray technicians. They are only required to disclose your files under subpoena.

Recovered addicts may be uneasy about confessing and discussing their history of addiction. But only when there is an honest and cooperative physician-patient relationship can the risks and benefits of medications be weighed, and the condition appropriately treated. Narcotic pain killers can spark a recovered addict's drug hunger and start the cycle all over again; forewarned, the physician can choose from among the new nonnarcotic pain killers. When the benefits of a drug outweigh its risks—as in the need for fentanyl in a complicated childbirth—the patient can be forewarned in time to gear up against the possible onset of drug hunger.

Open communication between patient and doctor is the best way to head off abuse and misuse and modify the staggering prescription drug abuse statistics. If your doctor is unwilling to discuss the pros and cons of drugs with you, is harsh or condescending once your use is revealed, or is unfamiliar with the latest knowledge about drugs, addiction, or dependency, consult another doctor. Find someone who knows at least as much as you do, sees drug abuse—not the drug abuser—as the problem, and is ready and waiting to help you with appropriate treatment.

Below we list your physician's duties and yours—and also those of your pharmacist.

Your Responsibilities:

- Know the generic names and brand names of the drugs you're taking.
- Tell the doctor who is giving you a prescription what other drugs you are using, including nonprescription drugs.
- Tell your doctor immediately if you become pregnant while taking drugs, or if you decide you want to become pregnant.
- Let your doctor know of any allergies you have experienced, however minor they may seem to you.
- Make sure you ask your doctor whether you can safely drink alcohol while taking the prescribed medicine.
- Ask whether the pills will have any effect on your ability to drive a car, or operate potentially dangerous machinery.
- Find out, by asking your doctor or pharmacist, whether you should avoid any specific foods or beverages while using the medicine.
- Follow instructions on dosage and schedule for the pills you're taking.
- Tell your doctor promptly if you think you're experiencing any adverse effects of the pills, or are suffering from some degree of overdose.
- If you believe you have had a major overdose, call for help or go immediately to the nearest emergency room for treatment. If possible, take with you the container the pills were in so hospital personnel can quickly identify the medicine involved and begin life-saving treatment without delay.

Your Doctor's Responsibilities:

- Your doctor should tell you exactly why the pills are being prescribed, that is, what your condition is and how the pills may help you.
- Your doctor should tell you what common side effects, such as headache, upset stomach, or sleepiness, can be expected from the pills.

- Your physician should also tell you what serious adverse effects, such as unusual heartbeat, difficulty breathing, unusual pains, or coma, may occur, and what to do if they do occur.
- Your doctor should be precise about how often to take the pills being prescribed, what dosage to take each time, and how long you should continue using the pills.
- You should be told whether any foods or beverages, especially alcohol, should be avoided while you're using the medicine.
- Your doctor should ask you detailed questions, perhaps through an assistant or by having you fill out a form, about your own and your family's medical history before prescribing any of the drugs described in this book or any other potentially dangerous drugs.
- Your physician should keep accurate, up-to-date records of every pill prescribed for you, and how often each prescription gets refilled.
- You should expect your doctor to spend as much time as is needed to answer questions about your medication.

Your Pharmacist's Responsibilities:

- The pharmacist filling your prescription must precisely follow the doctor's instructions written on the prescription form, and question the doctor if there is any doubt about the dosage or the medication.
- The pharmacist should be expected to answer questions you have about the pills you're getting, but cannot be expected to tell you why the doctor ordered the pills.
- The pharmacist should tell you what foods or beverages, if any, should be avoided while taking the pills, and whether the pills should be taken before, during, or after meals.
- The pharmacist should refuse to refill a prescription without authorization from the physician.

DRUG INTERACTIONS

Type of Drug	May Interact with:	To Produce:
Amphetamines	MAO inhibitors	hypertensive crisis (severe hypertension)
	antidepressants	more intense amphetamine reaction
	insulin	altered insulin requirements
	guanethidine sulfate	decreased antihypertensive effects
Methylphenidate hydrochloride	MAO inhibitors, antidepressants	increased effect of methylphenidate (may result in serious illness)
	guanethidine	decreased hypotensive effect
	anticoagulants, antidepressants, anticonvulsants, phenylbutazone, oxyphenbutazone	possible decrease in effectiveness of these drugs
Barbiturates	alcohol, antihistamines, other tranquilizers	increased sleepiness (may be fatal)
	anticoagulants, muscle relaxants, pain killers	decrease in effect of barbiturates and of other drugs
Ethchlorvynol	amitriptyline	delirium
	do *not* take with alcohol, antihistamines, other depressants	increased depressant effects
Methyprylon	antihistamines, alcohol, other depressants	increased sedative effects of methyprylon

DRUG INTERACTIONS

Type of Drug	May Interact with:	To Produce:
Methaqualone	alcohol, sleeping medications, antihistamines, tranquilizers, depressants	possible coma or death
Benzodiazepines	alcohol, tranquilizers, narcotics, sleeping pills, barbiturates, MAO inhibitors, antihistamines, antidepressants, depressants	very dangerous, even deadly effects
	cimetidine	possible prolonging of benzodiazepines' effects
	smoking	altered effectiveness of benzodiazepines (less drowsiness)
Carbamates	phenothiazines, tybamate and phenothiazines taken together	possible grand mal or petit mal seizures
	tranquilizers, alcohol, narcotics, barbiturates, sleeping pills, antihistamines, other depressants, antidepressants	excessive depression, sleepiness, fatigue
Hydroxyzine	alcohol, sedatives, tranquilizers, antihistamines, other depressants	increased drowsiness
Narcotic Analgesics	alcohol, sleeping medications, tranquilizers, other depressants	respiratory depression, hypotension, profound sedation, or coma
	use with care (and in reduced doses) with antihistamines, phenothiazines, antidepressants	increased depressant effects

DRUG INTERACTIONS

Type of Drug	May Interact with:	To Produce:
Antipsychotics	barbiturates, sleeping pills, narcotics, tranquilizers, other depressants, (alcohol)	increased depressant effects
	antidiarrheal mixtures, antacids	decreased phenothiazine effects
	guanethidine	inhibit antihypertensive action of guanethidine
Antidepressants	MAO inhibitors	high fevers, convulsions, even death
	oral contraceptives	possible decrease in effects of antidepressants
	ethchlorvynol (large doses)	possible delirium
	vitamin C (large doses), smoking	decrease in effectiveness of antidepressants
	alcohol	possible enhancement of effects of alcohol
	antihypertensives	decreased antihypertensive effects
	anticoagulants	increased anticoagulant effects
	sedatives	increased depressant effects
	thyroid medications	heart arrhythmias
	amphetamines	increased blood pressure

7
Pills and the Law

There may be as many laws—federal, state, and local—governing the manufacturing, distribution, sale, and use of pills, as there are brands, sizes, and shapes of the medications.

Federal agencies have traditionally taken the lead in attempting to halt pill abuse. A series of laws passed over the last 50 years has established criteria for defining dangerous drugs and set up enforcement agencies to help assure they are used only for medically approved purposes.

The main aim of federal drug control law has been to halt the traffic in narcotics, mainly heroin. But dozens of other drugs—including all the pills described in this book—are covered by federal, state, or local drug control laws.

The federal government in 1970 enacted the Controlled Substances Act (technically Title II, Comprehensive Drug Abuse Prevention and Control Act of 1970, Public Law 91-513), which took the place of several previous, sometimes inconsistent laws. The act established five categories, or "schedules," listing potentially abused medications. Prison terms and fines can follow violations in any schedule, but the harshest penalties are reserved for Schedules I and II, the least severe for Schedule V.

The 1970 law distinguishes between trafficking in controlled drugs and possessing them for personal use without a prescription or other approval. Trafficking is unauthorized manufacturing or distributing, or possession of a controlled drug with intent to distribute. Trafficking can bring a 30-year jail sentence and a $50,000 fine.

Conviction for illegal possession for personal use of a drug listed in any of the five schedules is a misdemeanor punishable by a one-year jail term and/or a $5000 fine for the first offense (or, if the violator is under 21, a possible year on probation followed by the destruction of all records of the conviction if the court approves), and penalties twice as severe for a subsequent offense.

Pharmacists are required to keep detailed records of the controlled drugs they dispense. Prescriptions must be kept on file, and inventories must be conducted at least every two years.

Decisions about which drugs belong in which schedule involve several agencies. The Drug Enforcement Agency and the Food and Drug Administration make preliminary evaluations and recommendations; then the DEA conducts hearings so that manufacturers and others can comment on the recommendations. If an administrative law judge drafts an order placing a drug in a schedule, the order becomes effective immediately.

Several factors must be considered before listing a drug or changing its schedule:

- evidence of the drug's effects on the mind or body;
- the state of current overall scientific knowledge about the drug;
- the drug's history and pattern of abuse;
- extent of abuse, i.e., whether abuse is a passing fad or widespread;
- risk to public health;
- extent of potential psychological or physical dependence; and
- whether the drug can easily be converted, in clandestine laboratories, to a drug already controlled by the 1970 law.

The government's five drug categories are:

SCHEDULE I

The drugs listed in Schedule I are the ones the government has determined have the highest potential for abuse. Usually they have no recognized medical use, except for experimental purposes. Substances include heroin and the hallucinogen LSD.

Extensive paperwork is required when Schedule I drugs are shipped. A special DEA document must be completed whenever the drugs change hands, and the government keeps close track of shipments and deliveries.

First offense penalties for trafficking in Schedule I drugs range from 5 years and $15,000 for a nonnarcotic drug to

15 years and $25,000 for a narcotic. Jail terms and fines are twice as severe for subsequent convictions.

Tight security is required at facilities making Schedule I drugs, including specially constructed vaults, alarm systems, and guards.

Since Schedule I drugs are almost always used within research institutions, there are no special prescription requirements.

SCHEDULE II

These drugs have legitimate medical uses, but possess a high potential for abuse. Most narcotics are listed in Schedule II, along with barbiturates and amphetamine compounds.

Extensive paperwork is also required when Schedule II drugs are shipped. Again, copies of a special DEA document must be completed.

Trafficking penalties are the same as those for Schedule I. Security requirements for manufacturers include specially constructed vaults, alarm systems, and guards.

Prescriptions for Schedule II drugs may be telephoned to a pharmacy only in an emergency, in which case the physician is required to provide the pharmacy with a written prescription within 72 hours. Prescriptions are void if not filled within six months. They may not be refilled.

SCHEDULE III

Drugs with moderate potential for abuse include nonbarbiturate sedatives, nonamphetamine stimulants (except cocaine, which is in Schedule II), and some narcotic preparations. Drugs in this category are viewed by the government as having the potential of leading to moderate or low physical dependence, or high psychological dependence.

Pharmacists and others who handle these drugs must maintain records that can be easily retrieved.

Penalties for trafficking in Schedule III drugs are five years and $15,000 for a first offense, and twice as long, or as much, for a subsequent conviction.

Security requirements are less strict: in lieu of a vault, for example, manufacturers may keep the drugs under surveillance in a secure area.

Prescriptions for Schedule III drugs can be telephoned to

a pharmacy by a physician, and can be refilled up to five times within six months, if the original prescription permits it.

SCHEDULE IV

Schedule IV drugs, which have less abuse potential than Schedule III drugs, and have limited likelihood of creating physical or psychological dependence, include some sedatives and several pain killers that do not contain narcotics.

Pharmacists and others who handle these drugs must maintain records that can be easily retrieved.

Penalties for trafficking are three years and $10,000 (first conviction), with penalties twice as severe for a subsequent conviction.

Security and prescription requirements are the same as for Schedule III substances.

SCHEDULE V

These drugs contain small amounts of narcotics and are used to control coughs and diarrhea. They have a low potential for abuse, and may lead to limited physical or psychological dependence.

Trafficking penalties are one year and $5000 fine (first offense), two years and $10,000 (subsequent).

Prescription requirements for many Schedule V drugs are the same as for Schedule III substances; however, many drugs in this group may be bought without prescription if the purchaser is at least 18 and can show identification. The purchaser's name is entered in a special log book maintained by the pharmacist and available for inspection by government drug control workers. Other record-keeping and security requirements are the same as for Schedule III drugs.

Prescriptions must be written in ink and include date of the prescription, full name and address of patient, and name, address, and DEA number of the physician who wrote the prescription.

The federal government has jurisdiction over importation into the United States and transportation across state lines of controlled drugs. Although drug violations within a state are state and local government concerns, there can be a federal role even if the drug has never crossed a state border. If a telephone is used, for example, the federal government may become involved because the phone is considered an interstate communications device.

State and local governments often have drug laws carrying even tougher penalties than federal laws. New York State enacted laws a few years ago that added years to the possible federal penalties and thousands of dollars to the fines.

To help you understand how drug laws apply to the pills discussed in this book, here are some often asked questions about pills, with answers drawn from the law and from the experience of those whose work concerns drugs, medicine, and the law.

QUESTIONS AND ANSWERS ABOUT PILLS AND THE LAW

Q: If a friend gives me some pills, say barbiturates, for which I don't have a prescription, am I breaking the law?

A: You can be charged with possession of controlled drugs if you are caught with them.

Q: If I pick up a prescription of narcotic pills for a friend who is too sick to go to the pharmacy, and I'm arrested for some reason before I deliver them to my friend, will I still be charged with possession?

A: You may be charged with possession, but the charge will almost certainly be dropped if you can demonstrate that your motives were innocent.

Q: If I'm taken to an emergency room with overdose symptoms, will the hospital notify anyone—my family, for instance, or the police—of my condition and what caused it?

A: The hospital will try to notify your family if permission is required for treatment and you are not in a condition to authorize it. Whether police are notified depends on what drug was involved in the overdose, whether it was accidental or a suicide attempt, and whether more drugs were found in your possession. Police and other drug control agencies are usually informed when narcotics are involved, but investigations usually don't go far unless there is evidence of crimes more serious than possession. Often, when an overdose victim is found to possess a large quantity of drugs, perhaps in pockets or among other personal effects, the drugs are simply disposed of by hospital workers after a sample is analyzed to make sure the patient is being treated correctly. The police prefer that the drugs be destroyed in their presence to assure they are not diverted to someone else.

Q: Can I be thrown out of school for popping pills?

A: Yes, in most school districts. Even if school authorities don't notify police or other officials about your use of pills, they can suspend or expel you from school under a variety of local statutes or regulations.

Q: If I am with a friend who is arrested for possession of pills just bought "on the street," can I be arrested too?

A: It is no crime to be with somebody who illegally possesses drugs. But police sometimes arrest everybody in a group when one member has drugs, and determine afterward who should or shouldn't be charged with a crime. This procedure is usually supported by courts. If you were present when your friend bought the drugs, however, you may be arrested and prosecuted for having taken part in the illegal purchase.

Q: If I am high on pills and collapse on the sidewalk, and a police officer searching my pockets to check my identity finds a dozen or more illegal pills in my pocket, will the search be considered illegal and the evidence be thrown out of court?

A: Such searches are often called good Samaritan searches, where the purpose is to help someone who appears to be in trouble. Courts consider contraband discovered in such a search as legally obtained; the pills can be introduced as evidence in court.

Q: I talked to some office colleagues about getting narcotics illegally, but didn't join their plan to steal or sell drugs. Can I be accused of any crime?

A: Yes, you might be charged with violating one of several conspiracy laws, even if you didn't participate in the final outcome of the conspiracy.

FEDERAL CLASSIFICATION OF CONTROLLED SUBSTANCES: (ABBREVIATED SCHEDULE)

Schedule I	Schedule II	Schedule III
Stimulants:	**Stimulants:**	**Stimulants:**
Amphetamine variants	Amphetamine	Benzphetamine
	Cocaine	Clortermine
Narcotic Analgesics:	Methamphetamine	Mazindol
Acetylmethadol	Methylphenidate	Phendimetrazine
(LAAM)	Phenmetrazine	
Heroin		**Sedatives/Depressants:**
	Sedatives/Depressants:	Any compound
Hallucinogens:	Amobarbital	containing an
Analogs of	Methaqualone*	unscheduled drug
phencyclidine	Pentobarbital	and amobarbital,
Ibogaine	Secobarbital	pentobarbital, or
Lysergic acid-25 (LSD)		secobarbital
Marijuana, hashish	**Narcotic Analgesics:**	Glutethimide
Mescaline	Alphaprodine	Methyprylon
Peyote	Anileridine	
Psilocybin, psilocyn	Codeine	**Narcotic Analgesics:**
Tetrahydrocannabinols	Dihydrocodeine	Acetaminophen +
	Ethylmorphine	Codeine
	Etorphine (M99)	APC + Codeine
	Fentanyl	Aspirin + Codeine
	Hydrocodone	Nalorphine
	Hydromorphone	Paregoric
	Levorphanol	
	Meperidine (pethidine)	
	Methadone	
	Morphine	
	Opium	
	Oxycodone	
	Oxymorphone	
	Phenazocine	
	Hallucinogens:	
	Phencyclidine	

Source: Bonnie Baird Wilford, *Drug Abuse, a Guide for the Primary Care Physician.* (Chicago: American Medical Association, 1981)

*Five states (Connecticut, Florida, Georgia, Mississippi, and New Jersey) classify methaqualone as a Schedule I drug.

Schedule IV	Schedule V
Stimulants: Diethylpropion Pemoline Phentermine **Sedatives/Depressants:** Barbital Chloral betaine Chloral hydrate Chlordiazepoxide Clonazepam Clorazepate Diazepam Ethchlorvynol Ethinamate Fenfluramine Flurazepam Mephobarbital Meprobamate Oxazepam Paraldehyde Pentazocine Phenobarbital Prazepam Propoxyphene Triazolam	Mixtures containing limited quantities of narcotic drugs, with nonnarcotic active medicinal ingredients. Less abuse potential than Schedule IV. Generally for antitussive and antidiarrheal pur- poses. May be distributed without a prescription order.

Q: Can a policeman search me for pills any time he wants to?

A: Certainly not. You cannot be searched unless you have been arrested, or have done something to clearly arouse the suspicions of the policeman. If you are in a car stopped for speeding or running a red light, you cannot be searched unless there is something clearly suspicious about the car or passengers (if it's a stolen car, for example). But if what appear to be drugs are in clear sight of the officer—on the car seat, for example—they can be confiscated, and a full search may legally follow.

Q: Under what circumstances can my teachers search me for drugs at school?

A: In general, teachers and school authorities have about the same rights as parents within the school facilities; but they will seldom subject students to a search unless there is a clear suspicion of drug usage. In some school districts, teachers and school administrators have a blanket authority to search desks and lockers whenever they wish.

Q. If I realize I'm hooked on pills, will I have to pay to get over my addiction?

A: If you need treatment quickly, you will probably have to pay a private clinic or doctor. While most areas have government-funded free clinics, most are understaffed, overcrowded, and underfunded. Some establish waiting lists, which can be months long, while others turn patients away without even taking their names (see pp. 87–91 for state-by-state list of drug abuse treatment programs).

Q: Can I be forced to participate in antidrug programs, or programs to stop addiction?

A: You cannot be "forced" to do so, but the alternatives made available to you—such as a jail sentence—may be so unpleasant that you will accept the option of a drug treatment program instead.

8
Lookalikes and Drugs of Deception

Lookalike drugs and drugs of deception are a recent but a growing part of the American drug-taking scene.

Lookalikes are tablets or capsules that resemble misused prescription drugs in shape, size, color, and/or markings, but do not contain the same ingredients or have the same effectiveness. The most common lookalikes are copies of amphetamine compounds, but instead of containing amphetamine, they contain caffeine, ephedrine, and/or phenylpropanolamine (PPA), an ingredient in many over-the-counter diet aid and decongestant products. These ingredients provide some stimulant effect but would be easily obtained without prescription, being available at much lower cost in a variety of products sold at supermarkets and drugstores.

Drugs of deception contain chemicals that require prescriptions when sold legally, but buyers can never be sure what chemicals they actually contain, and how much of each. A pill sold on the street as a barbiturate may really contain diazepam; another pill being pushed as amphetamine may contain a small amount of the amphetamine plus various untested ingredients.

The lookalike drug industry filled a vacuum inadvertently created by the 1970 Controlled Substances Act. The act (described in chapter 7) was the result of a growing recognition within the medical establishment and among lawmakers that existing laws had failed to adequately control drug abuse. The law created stiff penalties for illegal distribution of prescription drugs, but did not address misuse of nonprescription medications.

"Uppers" and "speed" had been widely misused in the preceding years, when they were frequently prescribed as appetite suppressants in weight control programs; for a rare condition known as narcolepsy, which causes its victims to suddenly fall asleep for brief periods throughout the day; and for children suffering from what has been called abnormal behavior syndrome or hyperactivity. (The amphetamine compounds are now recognized as having only limited usefulness to dieters.)

By then, amphetamine had been widely used for nearly a century. It first appeared in the late 19th century; by the 1930s amphetamine compounds were sold as decongestant inhalants, but they were soon used also as antidepressants, stimulants and appetite suppressants. During World War II they were given freely to Allied and Axis soldiers to relieve fatigue.

THE ERA OF DIET PILLS (1950–70)

Much of the early amphetamine trade was controlled by Smith Kline & French Laboratories, creators of such famous products as Dexedrine, Dexamyl, Eskatrol, and Benzedrine. The amphetamine market boomed in the late 1950s and early 1960s as America became obsessed with slimming down and staying thin.

It seemed for a while that almost everyone was taking the little black or pink pills that kept them from getting hungry. Middle-class students used the pills to stay awake while cramming for exams. Truck drivers carried sacks of "whites" during long-haul trips.

By the mid-1960s, more than 66,000 kilograms of amphetamine compounds were being manufactured every year in the United States. Fully half were diverted from legitimate wholesale supply channels to street corners, schoolyards, offices, and factories. Street buyers identified the products they wanted by shape and color: little pink or peach-colored triangular pills called "hearts"; sleek black capsules dubbed "black beauties"; and various speckled ones known as "Christmas trees."

Hip users knew the generic names and chemical classifications too, along with brand names like Desoxyn, Dexamyl, Obetrol, and the favorite for injection by "speed freaks," fast-acting methamphetamine.

Only after years of amphetamine use—and misuse—was it widely acknowledged that "uppers" have a dangerous down side. The drugs were being ground into powder and sniffed, or dissolved in water and injected. Psychological dependence and severe adverse effects were increasingly linked to high doses of amphetamine. Users were becoming more and more careless about dosage levels. Changes in perception caused by amphetamine led to many traffic deaths; the drugs created paranoia, with resultant suicide attempts; and violent crimes surrounding an amphetamine subculture increased dramatically. Establishment health officials and drug abuse specialists banded together to stem the soaring number of amphetamine abuse victims appearing in hospital emergency rooms.

GOVERNMENT STEPS IN

In 1970 the federal government took a strong stand on amphetamine. These drugs and some other stimulants were placed on Schedule II of the Controlled Substances Act, which lists drugs with a high potential for abuse and severely restricts their manufacture and distribution. The Food and Drug Administration immediately began limiting interstate shipments and banning imports from overseas. By 1972 the government had cut amphetamine production to less than 5 percent of what it had been a decade before.

One immediate effect of the new law was the birth of an underground industry producing poor-quality amphetamine for regular users. As manufacture of legitimate amphetamines plummeted, so did opportunities to steal or otherwise divert them from legal distribution systems. "Drugs of deception" and lookalikes became the replacement drugs of choice for many people turned on by stimulants.

The composition, purity, and potency of these "drugs of deception" are usually unknown to the user and vary from batch to batch. One pill bought "on the corner" may provide the desired high this week, but next week's supply may contain much less amphetamine, and three pills will be needed. Or the reverse may be true.

The potential for serious harm is apparent. If you're accustomed to popping a certain number of pills each day, and suddenly a much stronger supply comes along, you could become another overdose statistic at your local hospital emergency room—or coroner's office—without ever knowing why.

A scant 3 percent of all black market drugs of deception

contain any amphetamine whatsoever; the remaining 97 percent can also cause unexpected trouble. Without the quality control of legitimate manufacturing plants, the pills—with or without amphetamine—can and often do contain dangerous additives or impurities which cause severe reactions in susceptible users.

FAKE "SPEED" ON THE STREET

Reports of the "real stuff" being sold on the streets persisted and even escalated after the virtual outlawing of amphetamine in 1970. Drug clinics and government agencies continued hearing about black beauties, bennies, hearts, and dexies: Their prices had skyrocketed beyond the means of most users. (Now prices are low again because most users know that "blacks" are fake.)

Chemical analysis showed that much of the "speed" being pushed on the streets was some much milder stimulant like phendimetrazine, found in Plegine, or diethylpropion, used in Tepanil. These drugs were only listed in government's Schedule IV ("limited potential for abuse"). Their use as imitation "speed" has come under close FDA study, but they are not further restricted, in most states, and federal authorities do not consider stopping their sale on the street to be a law enforcement priority.

THE BIRTH OF LOOKALIKES

Even more of the street "amphetamine," analysis showed, contained no controlled drugs at all. This was the beginning of the lookalike drug market, which was to become a major industry with sales reported of almost $50 million in 1981.

According to some sources, it was William S. Saye, of Florida, who was the first to perceive a clear need among his fellow long-haul drivers for widely available, legal drugs to help them through long days and nights on the road. He obtained legal over-the-counter (nonprescription) diet aids and other caffeine-based stimulants from a New York drug manufacturer and sold them from his truck. Saye made good use of his CB radio, which most truckers install to warn each other of police speed traps. His CB handle was soon to become the newest nickname for the pills he sold: "Pea Shooter."

Within a few months the lookalike industry had spread across the nation. Manufacturers sprang up; students who couldn't obtain counterfeit speed containing a small amount of amphetamine or a similar drug spread the word about "legal speed." Lookalikes in a variety of shapes, colors, and strengths were suddenly being sold openly on college campuses, then through mail-order ads in magazines like *High Times* and *Penthouse,* and even at supermarket check-out counters.

The men and women marketing lookalike pills used clever sales promotions. Aware of the history of amphetamine, they made their pills in the image of their more powerful predecessors. "Black beauties" and "Christmas trees" were again widely sold, but this time with ingredients that anyone could buy at the local drugstore.

By 1980 more than 150 retail outlets and several mail-order establishments were known to be selling lookalikes which promised to curb appetite, eliminate fatigue, and be "100 percent safe." Advertising targets included not only the college-aged, but ever younger teens who were handed brochures at rock concerts and in their classrooms. Business cards were distributed by well-paid sales staffs.

The lookalike drugs contained, for the most part, a combination of phenylpropanolamine (PPA), ephedrine, and caffeine. PPA is an ingredient in over-the-counter diet aids such as Diadax, Dexatrim, and Dietac. (Note the similarities between the names of some nonprescription diet pills and the names of the all-but-banned amphetamine pills.)

By 1981 the size of the lookalike drug industry prompted federal authorities to take a closer look. A crackdown began, including FDA raids of manufacturing plants. Most raided pill-makers signed consent agreements to stop making the drugs in violation of several FDA regulations controlling their manufacturing and distribution, rather than endure long—and costly—court battles to stay in business.

But the lookalike industry didn't die. Some manufacturers went underground and continued their work in clandestine U.S. laboratories; their advertisements can still be found in a variety of publications.

Pricing of lookalike drugs is a problem. Since many people know that these illicit drugs are not the "real thing," buyers and sellers engage in extensive bargaining, and price wars periodically break out among sellers. The result so far seems to be an ever harder push by sellers to increase their profit line by selling more pills.

The attempt to destroy the multimillion-dollar lookalike drug industry, which sprang from the government's concern for the health and safety of its citizens, may have caused its emergence as a powerful underworld drug force. Some experts have suggested that the industry is likely to make more money after being driven underground. With newfound wealth and a vast market, some observers foresee the introduction of new stimulants created by the corporate descendants of a truck driver who wanted to stay awake while driving at night, and wanted his fellow truckers to do the same.

HOW SAFE ARE LOOKALIKE INGREDIENTS?

The physical effects of the ingredients commonly found in lookalike drugs are well known; their intensity depends on the amount ingested, and this can vary dramatically from maker to maker, and from pill to pill.

The most controversial ingredient is PPA. Ephedrine, considered by some experts to be the most dangerous, was cited by the FDA as the main reason for shutting down one large manufacturer in 1982. Caffeine may be the most habit forming of the ingredients, but because it is used so widely in our society, it is unlikely to be seriously restricted.

CAFFEINE

Caffeine stimulates the central nervous system throughout the brain and in the spinal column. The amount of caffeine in a typical lookalike pill ranges from 37 to 320 milligrams.

For comparison, a cup of coffee contains about 100 to 150 milligrams; a cup of tea, 60 to 75; a 12-ounce glass of a cola drink, 40 to 60. Experience indicates that 150 to 200 milligrams of caffeine is a safe dose for adults.

Precautions

Ulcers may be reactivated, and blood sugar levels increased, by caffeine use.

Common Side Effects

More than 200 milligrams of caffeine can result in nervousness, insomnia, and restlessness.

Severe Adverse Effects

Heart palpitations; nausea; impaired thinking; vomiting; rapid pulse; dizziness; stomach irritation; diarrhea; and muscular tremors. Doses of 500 milligrams or more may bring about extreme reactions resembling psychosis. Excessive urination can also occur.

Interactions

Birth control pills appear to interfere with the elimination of caffeine from the body, allowing higher concentrations to build up and leading to increased possibility of overdose.

Dependence and Addiction

Caffeine is widely recognized as habit forming. Excessive use may lead to tolerance and a mild withdrawal syndrome.

Withdrawal Symptoms

Headaches, depression, anxiety, and muscle weakness may be experienced after heavy caffeine usage is suddenly discontinued.

Withdrawal Treatment

Treatment of caffeine withdrawal is seldom required. The symptoms normally pass within a few days.

Overdose Symptoms and Treatment

Convulsions may occur if more than 10 grams (10,000 mg) of caffeine are consumed within a short period of time. Forcing the victim to vomit is usually the first stage of treatment, followed by psychological support from family, friends, and medical personnel.

Usage in Pregnancy

Excessive caffeine has been associated with premature births and increased fetal deaths. Birth defects have been noted in the offspring of laboratory rats fed high doses of caffeine. Pregnant women should avoid all products containing caffeine.

Usage During Breast Feeding

Not recommended. Caffeine appears in the breast milk of nursing mothers.

Usage by the Elderly

Tolerance to caffeine often decreases after 60. Side effects and adverse effects may be more pronounced.

Usage by Children

The dangers from caffeine are greater among children than among adults. Adults eliminate half the caffeine they consume within 4 hours, but infants take 4 to 6 days.

Dosage

Although the potentially lethal dose of caffeine is about 100 cups of coffee—that is, 30 or more powerful lookalike stimulant pills—users should remember that many products contain caffeine, and that high doses can be unknowingly accumulated.

EPHEDRINE

Ephedrine works by releasing a naturally occurring body chemical which acts as a central nervous system stimulant, causing the small blood vessels to contract and increasing blood pressure, heart rate, blood circulation, and metabolism.

Precautions

Anyone suffering from diabetes, prostatic problems, hypotension, angina pectoris, or chronic heart disease should not use ephedrine except under medical supervision. Some people are hypersensitive to this drug; you should avoid ephedrine if you have any reason to suspect you might be allergic to it.

Interactions

This drug may interfere with the ability of other drugs to reduce blood pressure. In combination with some other drugs—such as tricyclic antidepressants—ephedrine may cause large increases in blood pressure, which can lead to stroke.

Common Side Effects

Headaches and nervousness.

Serious Adverse Effects

Nausea; vomiting; insomnia; heart palpitations; tightness of the chest; sweating; and urinary problems.

Dependence and Addiction

A slight degree of tolerance may develop, but dependence and addiction are not known to occur.

Overdose Symptoms and Treatment

Symptoms of overdose can include the adverse effects listed above, in more extreme forms, along with muscle tremors. Toxic psychosis has occurred after long-term use of large doses. There is no specific treatment for the effects of overdose, other than overall medical support.

Usage in Pregnancy

This drug should be used with caution by pregnant women.

Usage During Breast Feeding

Not recommended. Traces of this drug are found in the breast milk of nursing mothers.

Usage by the Elderly

Small doses should be used until individual response has been determined, because of the sensitivity to this drug experienced by some elderly people.

Usage by Children

Children are more sensitive to this drug than adults, so use by children should be under medical supervision.

PHENYLPROPANOLAMINE (PPA)

This drug acts in a manner similar to ephedrine, resulting in stimulation of the central nervous system. The PPA content of a typical lookalike pill is 25 to 50 milligrams. Phenylpropanolamine, besides its stimulating effects, is used medically as a decongestant.

Precautions

Anyone with high blood pressure should use this drug with caution.

Interactions

PPA may increase the effects of epinephrine. It should not be used with MAO inhibitors or tricyclic antidepressants; such combinations may cause a dangerous increase in blood pressure.

Common Side Effects

Nervousness; insomnia; and increased blood pressure.

Serious Adverse Effects

Nausea; dizziness; anxiety; headache; muscle tremor; heart palpitations; and marked excitement.

Dependence and Addiction

There is no clear evidence that users become dependent on or addicted to PPA.

Overdose Symptoms and Treatment

A moderate overdose of PPA is marked by nervousness; restlessness; headache; heart palpitations; sweating; nausea; and vomiting.

A large overdose may cause extreme anxiety; confusion; delirium; muscle tremors; irregular pulse; and the threat of psychotic episodes. For some individuals, a large overdose can be fatal. Smaller overdoses have caused permanent heart damage and hypertension.

Treatment may consist of stomach pumping, forcing the victim to vomit or swallow activated charcoal, and use of a sedative like Valium.

Usage in Pregnancy

Not recommended.

Usage During Breast Feeding

Not recommended.

Usage by the Elderly

Only small doses should be used until individual sensitivity is established.

Usage by Children

Not recommended.

DO LOOKALIKES WORK?

The effectiveness of lookalike drug combinations is unclear. There has been little research into the combined effects of the stimulants caffeine, ephedrine, and PPA. Nor has there been adequate research comparing the effects of the lookalikes with the effects of real amphetamine compounds.

Probably effectiveness largely depends on individual sensitivity to the ingredients, along with nonmedical variables such as environment and others discussed in chapter 3. Most experienced drug users who take lookalikes say they experience a "mild buzz," or report: "They speed you up, but they're not speed."

Users, it appears, take lookalike stimulants to achieve the mood, not the total physical response, of amphetamines. They assume that lookalikes are safe and weak substances. They don't realize that dosage also determines impact, and that large doses can be dangerous.

The safety of lookalikes depends on your age, weight, and general tolerance. Side effects can range from sleep

disturbances to psychotic episodes. With lookalike ingredients available from so many sources, the chance of unin-
tentional overdose *may* be more likely than with genuine
amphetamines. Since the proportion of the ingredients keeps
changing, users' physical and emotional reactions are
unpredictable.

LOOKALIKE OVERDOSES

During the heyday of amphetamines, "Speed Kills" took
on a meaning beyond that of auto safety. Lately, about a
dozen deaths from lookalike stimulants have been reported,
ushering in a new era with the slogan "Fake Speed Kills."

Medical experts report that three to four times the usual
dosage of a lookalike drug can cause symptoms of overdose.
An overdose of PPA alone—known as "being overamped"—
is usually treated by making the victim vomit and then
swallow activated charcoal, which prevents some of the
drug still in the stomach from being digested. A sedative
like Valium may be used to treat the victim's anxiety.

Another danger of a lookalike overdose is elevated blood
pressure, for which an antihypertensive drug may have to
be provided intravenously. Within a few hours the lookalike
ingredients will be excreted with the urine; until then,
symptoms such as hallucinations are dealt with by keeping
the victim calm and offering reassurance that the discomfort will soon pass.

An added danger of lookalike overdose is that emergency room staffs cannot treat the victim with full effectiveness because they have no way of knowing what doses of
each ingredient in the pills have been taken.

It is certain that new lookalike substances will appear on
the streets. The main criterion will be that they meet consumer demand—not that they are safe. The following table,
provided by *Drug Survival News*, lists some forms and
contents of lookalike stimulants as they exist today. The
chart could well be titled "Let the Buyer Beware."

LOOKALIKES ANALYSIS

	DRUG CONTENT		
Description and Markings	Caffeine (mg.)	Ephedrine (mg.)	Phenylpro-panolamine (mg.)
Tablets:			
Pink, heart shape	106 200	12.5 25	36.7 50
Pink, oval shape ("pink footballs")	98.1 150 200	15.8 50 50	— 25 25
White, oblong shape, green specks	46.8 176.4 200	22.3 12.6 25	— — 50
White, round shape, one cross ("whites")	—	25	25
Orange, round shape, imprinted "BT 72"	175	25	37.5
Blue, and dark blue/white specks	150	50	25
White, oblong shape, blue specks	200 175	25 25	50 50
Capsules:			
Brown and clear capsule, white and orange granules, imprinted "127"	37.1 173.2 25	16.6 — 25	45.3 — 50
White and clear capsule, white, orange, and green granules, imprinted "127"	110.9 200	26.6 25	61.2 —
Green and clear capsule, white and green granules, imprinted "127" ("Christmas tree speed")	137.9 323.8 200	13.4 — —	58.2 — 30

LOOKALIKES ANALYSIS

DRUG CONTENT

Description and Markings	Caffeine (mg.)	Ephedrine (mg.)	Phenylpro-panolamine (mg.)
Capsules (cont.):			
Black and clear capsule, imprinted "18-845," "18-858," "17-875"	180 100	2.2 25	46.5 50
Yellow capsule, imprinted "RJ8," "RUS," "RJS," "18-906"	200 100 125 100	25 25 25 25	50 50 37.5 50
Black capsule, imprinted "RJS" ("black beauties") "DEX," "127"	125 200 200	25 25 25	50 50 50
Black capsule, white powder, brown and black granules, imprinted "18-789," "RUS"	172.1 125 44.5	9.0 25 —	— 50 2.1
Black capsule, white powder, black pellets, imprinted "335"	200 144.4	25 24.5	50 55.1

Information obtained from street drug analysis reports or supplied by manufacturers and distributors. Courtesy of *Drug Survival News,* May-June 1981, D.I.N. Publications/Do It Now Foundation.

II

The Most Commonly Prescribed Psychoactive Drugs in the United States, Generic, Brand, and Street Names, with Complete Profiles of Drugs and Their Effects

1. Stimulants

Amphetamine

Amphetamine Combination

Amphetamine Complex

Amphetamine Mixtures

Amphetamine Sulfate

Dextroamphetamine Sulfate

Methamphetamine
Hydrochloride

Other Stimulants

Methylphenidate
Hydrochloride

Pemoline

A substantial percentage of stimulants commonly available in pill form, whether by prescription or through illicit street purchases, are amphetamine compounds—commonly known as "speed" or "uppers"—or chemicals purported to produce similar effects: some degree of euphoria, and an ability to stay awake for long periods.

The underground use of amphetamine has been overshadowed in recent years by the renewed popularity of another stimulant, cocaine, first used a century ago as a local anesthetic in nose and throat surgery.

But the demand for amphetamine remains high. When amphetamine itself is hard to get in the illegal drug marketplace, other preparations are sold in its place. Over the past few years, amphetamine compounds have been increasingly replaced by "lookalike" stimulants, pills carefully molded into shapes nearly identical to the most popular amphetamine pills but actually containing such nonprescription drugs as caffeine and phenylpropanolamine (PPA). A brief history of the lookalike drug industry, and descriptions of what lookalike pills really contain, can be found in chapter 8.

Among the first modern stimulants to be commercially produced was ephedrine, which comes from the Chinese herb *Ephedra vulgaris*. For centuries the plant has been used in traditional oriental medicine for treatment of bronchial conditions; it expands the bronchial muscles, constricts blood vessels and mucous membranes, and raises blood pressure. Once the principal active ingredient, ephedrine, was isolated at the beginning of the 20th century, researchers learned that in sufficient doses it can also produce a dramatic decrease in the muscle movements throughout the digestive system.

But ephedrine caused serious side effects in large numbers of people using it, and adequate supplies of the herb were difficult to obtain. A search began for a safer, easily produced substitute. In the 1920s researcher Gordon Alles created a synthetic replacement, amphetamine, which was initially believed to have few side effects.

Other modern stimulants soon followed. Some of those pills have amphetaminelike properties but are chemically different from amphetamine, including methylphenidate hydrochloride (Ritalin) and pemoline (Cylert), both prescribed to treat abnormal behavior syndrome in children. They are considered by many to be less harmful than amphetamine compounds, and Ritalin remains popular among stimulant pill abusers.

AMPHETAMINE

Amphetamine has been a significant part of America's drug scene for more than half a century. While today the drug's use in helping people lose weight has greatly diminished, it remains a medically accepted mode of treatment for abnormal behavior syndrome in children, and narcolepsy.

In the mid-1930s, shortly after amphetamine was purified in a San Francisco laboratory, it was widely sold throughout the U.S. without prescription in the form of small, portable inhalants to relieve bronchial spasms and nasal congestion. At the time amphetamine was produced only as a liquid, and the inhalants were filled with absorbent materials permeated with the drug. These inhalants were used regularly by those seeking their stimulant effects: white-collar workers trying to stretch their days, housewives hoping to feel their best when their husbands came home, factory laborers seeking to increase alertness while performing difficult tasks.

Soon after amphetamine became available in tablets, the drug's use skyrocketed. Pills were regularly issued to servicemen and prescribed to civilians in a way that would be regarded today as careless and irresponsible.

Soldiers were issued amphetamine so they would have a better chance of survival on the battlefield during World War II. Fighter pilots on long missions made widespread use of the drug, as did those forced to remain in a state of combat readiness for extended periods. The drug was used by German and Japanese military personnel, as well as British and American. At the time, however, amphetamine was seen as a safe, effective remedy against sleepiness, and was prescribed for a wide range of other complaints.

By the 1960s researchers began to recognize that amphetamine preparations carried risks, and that other, more effective ways were available to treat many of the conditions for which amphetamine was being prescribed.

State and federal officials took their first tentative steps toward controlling the nationwide use of amphetamine preparations; beginning in 1965 their small steps became huge strides once hospitals began identifying the preparations as the cause of serious overdoses, many of them resulting in a condition called amphetamine psychosis, which often mimicked classical paranoid schizophrenia. Resulting legislation in the late 1960s curtailed the prescription of these drugs, and illegal use increased greatly.

Although recently there has been a considerable reduction in the illicit use of these drugs, they are still popular among those seeking the initial euphoria amphetamine preparations can provide. While the most intense exhilaration comes from injected drugs, which take effect in just a few minutes, many individuals prefer the slightly slower effects that stem from pills.

Amphetamine compounds (especially methamphetamine, which is highly soluble) are, however, frequently dissolved in water and injected to produce a sensation users describe as total-body orgasm. Known as a "flash" or "rush," the sensation quickly disappears. To maintain it, amphetamine enthusiasts will engage in "speed runs," during which they inject a new dose every hour or so.

After the "run" begins, users usually experience an intense desire to talk endlessly. A few injections later, though, they are likely to face persecution fantasies and illusions. When exhaustion takes hold and the user "crashes" from his high level of exhilaration, he may sleep for up to two days and nights, then wake up extremely hungry. Suicidal tendencies and depression are common in frequent users during the periods between "speed runs."

Several amphetamine compounds are sold by a number of drug manufacturers, all chemically so alike as to make them indistinguishable except by laboratory analysis. Their differences stem from the variety of their dosages, and slight structural alterations which vary the way in which they are metabolized.

Amphetamine pills begin to affect the central nervous system within about 30 minutes, causing elevation of blood pressure, rapid breathing, and overall stimulation. The drugs work for up to about 14 hours. They slow digestive system muscles, thus reducing appetite. Because of this effect, for about a decade amphetamine compounds were frequently prescribed to aid weight loss. Sometimes doctors injected the drug; more often they prescribed pills, renewing the prescriptions even when their patients failed to demonstrate results. There is intense debate in medical circles about this use. Some states have severely restricted the use of amphetamine in dietary programs; a few have completely banned such use.

It is tempting to compare the use of amphetamine a decade or so ago to the modern proliferation of diet plans—some including medications to diminish appetite—which number in the dozens. Future years will show whether a dark side is to be found in today's diet "miracles."

Amphetamine and amphetaminelike substances (such as Fastin and Ionamin) are suggested for use nowadays in aiding weight loss only in cases of extreme obesity, when repeated diets and other therapies have failed. Such use, according to current medical thinking, should be limited to two to four weeks, after which tolerance to the drugs develops and they lose effectiveness for weight loss. Other accepted amphetamine uses include treatment of abnormal behavior syndrome in children (also called hyperactivity), when amphetamine is part of a treatment program including psychological, social, and educational assistance.

Amphetamine compounds are also prescribed for narcolepsy, a condition causing its victims to suddenly fall asleep, usually for brief periods, frequently during the day.

It is little wonder that amphetamine is popularly known as "speed." Among those using these drugs for recreational reasons, the most frequent aims are to speed up mental ability, struggle against fatigue, and gain a sensation of increased strength and sexuality. Recent research indicates that small doses of amphetamine may in fact enhance sexual performance in people suffering from certain sexual ailments, but that high doses seriously impair sexual functioning.

Precautions

Do not use these drugs if you have any reason to suspect you are allergic to any of the amphetamine compounds. Some amphetamine pills contain tartrazine, which may cause serious reactions (including bronchial asthma) in susceptible individuals, often those who are allergic to aspirin.

Because these drugs may cause dizziness and mask extreme fatigue, you should be careful if you are driving, operating potentially dangerous machinery, or performing some other task that requires concentration or alertness.

Do not use these drugs if you suffer from advanced arteriosclerosis, heart disease, moderate to severe hypertension, hyperthyroidism, or glaucoma; or if you have a history of drug abuse.

Interactions

Do not use amphetamine compounds if you have used MAO inhibitor drugs within the preceding two weeks: a hypertensive crisis may result. Do not use amphetamine with tricyclic antidepressants; the combination will cause a more intense amphetamine reaction.

Among diabetes sufferers, insulin requirements may be altered by the use of amphetamine.

Amphetamine may decrease the effects of some drugs used to treat high blood pressure, especially guanethidine sulfate.

Common Side Effects

Nervousness; restlessness; insomnia; dizziness; lack of appetite; dry mouth; and various digestive difficulties.

Serious Adverse Effects

Palpitations; tachycardia; elevation of blood pressure; overstimulation; involuntary headache; psychotic episodes; unpleasant taste; diarrhea; constipation; and anorexia.

Loss of appetite and weight loss may occur as undesirable adverse effects when amphetamine is used for purposes other than weight reduction.

Impotence and loss of sexual desire have been reported during periods of heavy amphetamine use.

Dependence and Addiction

Extreme psychological dependence occurs with frequent overuse of amphetamine. While tolerance develops in two to four weeks, there is some doubt among researchers about whether actual physical dependence develops.

Symptoms of chronic usage of amphetamine may include severe skin rash; insomnia; irritability; hyperactivity; personality changes; and hypertension.

More severe symptoms associated with high dosage levels may include a psychosis clinically identical to schizophrenia.

Withdrawal Symptoms

Extreme fatigue and mental depression may occur when these drugs are abruptly stopped, especially after using high dosages.

Although no life-threatening symptoms of withdrawal have been observed, regular heavy users may experience suicidal tendencies between doses.

Withdrawal Treatment

Amphetamine withdrawal is usually handled by medical personnel by close observation and continual reassurance that the severe symptoms of depression and lethargy will diminish. Valium is sometimes administered.

Overdose Symptoms and Treatment

The amount of amphetamine required to produce serious overdose symptoms depends to a large extent on the frequency of previous usage and the size of the doses. The lethal dose is many times as high as the dose needed for therapeutic or recreational effects, and after repeatedly taking amphetamine, most people develop high tolerance to the drug. One man swallowed twenty 5 mg. tablets and recovered with no ill aftereffects within three days. Another, after ingesting 28 such tablets, died of acute kidney failure, fever, jaundice, and circulatory collapse.

Symptoms of amphetamine overdose include restlessness; tremor; hostile mood swings; confusion; rapid breathing; hallucinations; and panic.

Cardiovascular symptoms include arrhythmias; hypertension or hypotension; and circulatory collapse.

Gastrointestinal symptoms may include nausea; vomiting; diarrhea; and abdominal cramps. Fatal overdoses are usually preceded by convulsions and coma. Anyone suspected of having taken an amphetamine overdose must be taken to a hospital immediately. Always bring the pill bottle so the emergency room staff can identify the medication and begin proper treatment without delay.

Amphetamine overdose will be treated differently depending on the amount of the drug taken and the victim's tolerance level.

A generally nontolerant victim may be treated with diazepam (Valium) pills and reassurance, a technique known as "supportive and symptomatic." A more serious overdose may require antipsychotic medication—like Thorazine or Haldol—or Valium delivered intravenously.

Stomach pumping is used only within the first hour after overdose.

Usage in Pregnancy

Not recommended.

Usage During Breast Feeding

Traces of these drugs may be present in the breast milk of nursing mothers, so their use should be weighed against the possible adverse effects on infants.

Usage by the Elderly

Normal adult doses permitted.

Usage by Children

Not recommended for weight control in children under 12. Not recommended for any reason in children under 3.

Generic Name

Amphetamine Combination (Schedule II)

Brand Name (and Company)

Eskatrol (SKF)

Ingredients

Dextroamphetamine Sulfate (15 mg.)
Prochlorperazine Maleate (an antipsychotic) (7.5 mg.)

Most Commonly Prescribed for

Weight reduction

General Information

Eskatrol is no longer manufactured, but supplies may still be available and some physicians may continue to prescribe the drug.

Dosage

1 capsule in the morning
Available size: 22.5 mg. capsules.

Important: Precautions and warnings about this drug, pp 126–131

Generic Name

Amphetamine Complex (Schedule II)

Brand Name (and Company)

Biphetamine (Pennwalt)

Ingredients

Amphetamine
Dextroamphetamine

Street Name

Blacks.

Most Commonly Prescribed for

Weight reduction; abnormal behavior syndrome in children.

Dosage

ADULTS
  Obesity: 12.5 to 20 mg. total daily taken early in the day.
CHILDREN (6–12)
  Abnormal behavior syndrome: 5 to 10 mg. total daily divided into 1 to 2 doses gradually increased each week until results are ideal.

CHILDREN (3–5)
Abnormal behavior syndrome: 2.5 mg. total daily gradually increased until results are ideal.
Available sizes: 12.5 and 20 mg. capsules.

Important: Precautions and warnings about this drug, pp 126–131

Generic Name

Amphetamine Mixtures (Schedule II)

Brand Names (and Companies)

Amphaplex (Vortech)
Delcobese (Delco)
Obetrol (Obetrol)

Ingredients

Salts of Amphetamine and Dextroamphetamine in various amounts

Most Commonly Prescribed for

Weight reduction; abnormal behavior syndrome in children; narcolepsy.

Dosage

ADULTS
Narcolepsy: 5 to 60 mg. total daily in divided doses.
Weight reduction: 5 to 30 mg. total daily in divided doses 30 to 60 minutes before meals (or a long-acting form once in morning).
CHILDREN (6–12)
Abnormal behavior syndrome: 5 to 10 mg. total daily divided into 1 to 2 doses gradually increased each week until results are ideal.
CHILDREN (3–5)
Abnormal behavior syndrome: 2.5 mg. total daily gradually raised each week until results are ideal.
Available sizes: 5, 10, 15, and 20 mg. tablets; 5, 10, and 15 mg. capsules.

Important: Precautions and warnings about this drug, pp 126–131

Generic Name

Amphetamine Sulfate (Schedule II)

Brand Names (and Companies)

Amphetamine Sulfate (Lannett)
Benzedrine (SKF)
Benzedrine Spansules (SKF)

Street Names

Bennies; peaches; splash; crystal; crank; meth; speed; water; beans; black beauties; black Cadillacs; black mollies; brown and clears; crosses; crossroads; double cross; hearts; minibennies; pep pills; rosas; roses; thrusters; truck drivers; uppers; wake-ups; whites.

Most Commonly Prescribed for

Weight reduction; abnormal behavior syndrome in children; narcolepsy.

Dosage

ADULTS
  Narcolepsy: 5 to 60 mg. total daily in divided doses.
  Weight reduction: 5 to 30 mg. total daily in divided doses 30 to 60 minutes before meals (or a sustained-release form once in morning).
CHILDREN (6–12)
  Abnormal behavior syndrome: 5 to 10 mg. total daily divided into 1 to 2 doses gradually increased each week until results are ideal.
CHILDREN (3–5)
  Abnormal behavior syndrome: 2.5 mg. total daily gradually increased each week until results are ideal.
Available sizes: 5 and 10 mg. tablets; 15 mg. sustained-release capsules.

Important: Precautions and warnings about this drug, pp 126–131

Generic Name

Dextroamphetamine Sulfate (Schedule II)

Brand Names (and Companies)

Dexedrine (SKF)   Robese (Rocky Mountain)
Dexampex (Lemmon)   Spancap (North American)
Ferndex (Ferndale)   Tidex (Allison)
Oxydess (North American)
Also sold under generic name

Street Names

Copilots; dexies; oranges; footballs.

Most Commonly Prescribed for

Weight reduction; abnormal behavior syndrome in children; narcolepsy.

Dosage

ADULTS

Narcolepsy: 5 to 60 mg. total daily in divided doses. Should not be taken within 6 hours of bedtime.

Weight reduction: 5 to 10 mg. total daily in divided doses 30 to 60 minutes before meals (or sustained-release form once in morning).

CHILDREN (6–12)

Abnormal behavior syndrome: 5 to 10 mg. total daily divided into 1 to 2 doses, gradually increased each week until results are ideal (or sustained-release form once daily).

CHILDREN (3–5)

Abnormal behavior syndrome: 2.5 mg. total daily gradually increased each week until results are ideal.

Important: Precautions and warnings about this drug, pp 126–131

Generic Name

Methamphetamine Hydrochloride
(Schedule II)

Brand Names (and Companies)

Desoxyn (Abbott)
Desoxyn Gradumets (Abbott)
Methampex (Lemmon)

Street Names

Crystal; meth; speed.

Most Commonly Prescribed for

Weight reduction; abnormal behavior syndrome in children.

Precautions

15 mg. sustained-release tablets contain tartrazine, which
may cause allergic reactions in those sensitive to aspirin.

Dosage

ADULTS
   Weight reduction: 5 mg. 30 minutes before every meal
(or 10 to 15 mg. sustained-release form before breakfast).
CHILDREN
   Abnormal behavior syndrome: 5 to 10 mg. total daily
divided into 1 to 2 doses, gradually increased every week
until response is ideal.
Available sizes: 5 and 10 mg. tablets; 5, 10, and 15 mg.
sustained-release tablets.

Important: Precautions and warnings about this drug, pp 126–131

OTHER STIMULANTS

Generic Name

Methylphenidate Hydrochloride (Schedule II)

Brand Names (and Companies)

Ritalin (Ciba)
Also sold under generic name

Street Names

West coast; pellets.

Most Commonly Prescribed for

Abnormal behavior syndrome in children; narcolepsy.

General Information

Methylphenidate has a stimulant effect similar to amphetamine, but is chemically different. Its main advantage over amphetamine compounds appears to be a reduction in dangerous side effects.

Although this drug works as a stimulant in most people, it has the opposite effect in children with short attention spans, emotional instability, or moderate to severe hyperactivity. They appear to be calmed down by methylphenidate, and frequently do much better in school. The children themselves report that they feel "changed" by the drug, but not sedated. There is, however, an intense debate among physicians and researchers on whether the drug should be used in this way, since it is questionable whether basic behavior patterns are altered by methylphenidate. For this reason, physicians generally use this drug in conjunction with counseling, psychotherapy, and other behavior-modifying treatments.

Precautions

Do not take methylphenidate if you are extremely tense or agitated; if you have glaucoma; if you have high blood pressure; or if you have a history of seizures.

Do not take this drug if you have any reason to think you may be allergic to it.

Since methylphenidate may cause dizziness, be careful if you are driving, operating potentially dangerous machinery, or performing some other task that requires concentration and alertness.

Interactions

Methylphenidate will decrease the effectiveness of guanethidine, a drug used to treat high blood pressure.

Interaction with MAO inhibitor drugs, and with tricyclic antidepressants, may vastly increase the effect of methylphenidate and cause very serious illness.

This drug should be used cautiously with anticoagulants (blood-thinning drugs); many medications used to treat convulsions; phenylbutazone; oxyphenbutazone; and antidepressant drugs.

Common Side Effects

The most common side effects in adults include nervousness and insomnia. Children frequently experience loss of appetite; stomach pains; weight loss; and sleeping difficulty.

Serious Adverse Effects

Occasional: skin rash; itching; fever; symptoms similar to arthritis; nausea; dizziness; abnormal heart rhythms; headache; drowsiness; changes in blood pressure or pulse; chest pains; stomach pains; psychotic reactions; changes in blood composition; and loss of hair. A child's growth rate may be slowed by this drug.

Dependence and Addiction

Although a relatively safe drug when used under close medical supervision, methylphenidate has been widely misused by adults seeking its stimulant effects. Such misuse often leads to psychological dependence. Varying types of unusual behavior—including fidgeting and excitability—may be signs of misuse.

Withdrawal Symptoms

Suddenly stopping the use of this drug can lead to severe depression.

Withdrawal Treatment

Treatment of withdrawal from methylphenidate, which should be supervised by a physician, usually includes gradually reducing the dosage over a period of several days, while at the same time providing reassurance that the depression will soon pass.

Overdose Symptoms and Treatment

Vomiting; agitation; tremor; euphoria; confusion; hallucinations; delirium; sweating; flushing of the face, hands, and extremities; severe headache; high fever; abnormal heart rate; high blood pressure; dryness of the mouth and nose; and convulsions followed by coma.

Anyone suspected of having taken a methylphenidate overdose must be rushed to a hospital immediately. Always bring the pill bottle so the emergency room staff can quickly identify the medication and begin treatment without delay.

Treatment for a methylphenidate overdose usually includes protecting the victim from injuring himself, and keeping him from being exposed to loud voices, bright lights, and other external stimuli that may aggravate the overstimulation already present. Stomach pumping is sometimes required, preceded by a dose of a slow-acting barbiturate. If the overdose is severe, medical personnel may undertake a variety of measures to assure that blood circulation and breathing remain adequate.

Usage in Pregnancy

Not recommended.

Usage During Breast Feeding

Safety has not been established.

Usage by the Elderly

The smallest effective doses may be used.

Usage by Children

The long-term effects of this drug on children have not
been determined. Periodic "drug holidays," when the drug
is temporarily suspended, are urged. Not recommended
for children under 6.

Dosage
ADULTS

Narcolepsy: 20 to 30 mg. total daily divided into 2 to 3
doses taken 30 minutes before meals (rarely up to 60 mg.
total daily in divided doses).

CHILDREN (over 6 through early puberty)

Abnormal behavior syndrome: 10 to 20 mg. total daily
divided into 2 doses (before breakfast and lunch) gradually
increased to maximum 60 mg. total daily in divided doses.
Available sizes: 5, 10, and 20 mg. tablets.

Generic Name

Pemoline (Schedule IV)

Brand Name (and Company)

Cylert (Abbott)

Most Commonly Prescribed for

Abnormal behavior syndrome in children.

General Information

Cylert is a central nervous system stimulant structurally
different from amphetamine and methylphenidate. It is
not known why it works in children with abnormal behavior syndrome or attention deficit disorders.

Although Cylert is not as well known as the other
stimulants, it can still be bought on the street, where it is
sometimes sold as "safe speed." Research shows that it
has few, if any, adverse reactions with other drugs, and its
undesirable effects are considered somewhat milder than
those experienced with many other stimulants.

Precautions

Don't use Cylert if you have any reason to suspect you are allergic to it.

This drug should be used cautiously by people with kidney or liver ailments.

Because dizziness and drowsiness can occur, be careful if you are driving, operating potentially dangerous machinery, or performing some other task that requires concentration and alertness.

Interactions

No serious interactions with other drugs are known.

Common Side Effects

Insomnia; loss of appetite (anorexia); stomachache; headache; irritability; rash; mild depression; dizziness; and drowsiness.

Serious Adverse Effects

Involuntary movements of the tongue, lips, face, hands, and feet; and wandering eye are possible. Seizures have been reported after usage, but have not been directly tied to Cylert. Hallucinations have also occurred.

Dependence and Addiction

Psychological and/or physical dependence may occur with this drug.

Withdrawal Symptoms

Depression is the main symptom of Cylert withdrawal.

Withdrawal Treatment

Treatment of withdrawal depression, which should be handled by qualified medical personnel, usually includes gradually reducing the dosage while providing psychological support.

Overdose Symptoms and Treatment

Rapid heartbeat; hallucinations; agitation; uncontrolled

muscle movements; extreme restlessness; irregular breathing; increased salivation; and occasional tongue protrusions. Psychotic symptoms may occur. Anyone suspected of having taken a Cylert overdose must be rushed to a hospital. Always bring the pill bottle so the emergency room staff can properly identify the drug and begin appropriate treatment without delay.

Treatment may include stomach pumping, sedation, and other supportive measures.

Usage in Pregnancy

Not recommended.

Usage During Breast Feeding

Not recommended.

Usage by the Elderly

Not recommended.

Usage by Children

Permitted in children over 6 within doses outlined below. Children should be closely monitored for any changes in their growth rate while taking this drug. Psychotic children may experience worsening of their symptoms during Cylert therapy.

Dosage

CHILDREN (over 6)

Abnormal behavior syndrome: 37.5 mg. total daily in 1 morning dose gradually increased to maximum 112.5 mg. total daily in 1 morning dose.
Available sizes: 18.75, 37.5, and 75 mg. tablets.

2. Sedatives

Barbiturates

Amobarbital and
   Amobarbital Sodium
Barbital
Butabarbital Sodium
Hexobarbital
Mephobarbital
Metharbital

Pentobarbital and
   Pentobarbital Sodium
Phenobarbital
Secobarbital and
   Secobarbital Sodium
Talbutal

Barbiturate Combinations

Butatrax
Butseco
Carbrital Kapseals
Ethobral
Hyptran
Lull
Nidar
Penotal

Plexonal
Quan III
S.B.P.
Secanap
Secophen
Tri-Barbs
Tuinal Pulvules
Twinbarbital #2

Barbituratelike Sedatives

Chloral Hydrate
Ethchlorvynol
Glutethimide

Methaqualone
Methyprylon

Benzodiazepines

Alprazolam
Chlordiazepoxide
   Hydrochloride
Clorazepate Dipotassium
Diazepam
Flurazepam Hydrochloride

Halazepam
Lorazepam
Oxazepam
Prazepam
Temazepam
Triazolam

Benzodiazepinelike Sedatives

Carbamates
Meprobamate
Tybamate

Hydroxyzine
Hydroxyzine Hydrochloride
   and Hydroxyzine Pamoate

Sedatives have been used for thousands of years. Ancient writings are filled with references to various naturally occurring substances, most often plants, which when eaten or drunk in liquid potions either eased anxiety or caused sleep. Understandably, those who knew which plants, and in what dosages, produced the desired effects had a great deal of power over wealthy insomniacs and anxiety-ridden authorities. Even religious writings refer to the use of unnamed substances with sedative properties. Samson, at Delilah's request, was presumably given a sleeping potion while his hair was cut—and his powers lost.

Yet until the 19th century there was little understanding of how sedatives worked. Nor is the precise way they function clearly understood, even today, after decades of complex laboratory analysis and studies of thousands of people who have used modern sedatives under medical supervision.

An estimated 20 million Americans suffer from recurring insomnia, according to experts, and another 100 million experience temporary inability to sleep during a family crisis, the loss of a job, the dying of a loved one, or some other difficulty. The majority of such people seek help from physicians, who usually prescribe sleeping pills. Current medical opinion indicates that sedatives are most effective for such temporary insomnia, rather than for long-standing difficulties in falling asleep.

Sedatives in common use today can be divided into barbiturates and nonbarbiturates. The barbiturates include widely abused drugs like Nembutal or Seconal, also known by street names such as "yellow jackets" and "nebbies." The nonbarbiturate sedatives, also widely abused, include the popular family of drugs known as benzodiazepines, among them Librium and Valium as well as several important but less well-known compounds.

Both classes of sedatives are dangerous if not used strictly under medical supervision. Most sedatives are potentially addictive—physically, psychologically, or both—and may cause serious injury or death if taken in sufficiently large doses, or in combination with other drugs or alcohol. They should be approached with caution by consumers concerned about their well-being, and used, if at all, as conservatively as possible.

Some physicians and researchers insist on classifying

the individual drugs as sedatives or hypnotics—from the Greek word *hypnotikos*, to put to sleep—apparently believing that some of them will only calm you down, while others will make you sleepy. But the effects of all appear to be "dose-related," that is, a small dose will calm you down, while a sufficiently large dose will make you fall asleep. Some, however, are used for only one purpose or the other, depending on the drug's potency, dose-related dangers, and the way they were marketed by the manufacturers.

BARBITURATES

Barbiturates, first used medically in 1882, stem from the combination of urea—the main nonliquid component of urine—and malonic acid, which comes from apples. This unusual compound was developed, for reasons now lost to history, by the German chemist Adolph Baeyer in 1865.

Whether barbiturates take their name from a Munich waitress named Barbara, who contributed urine samples for analysis, or from St. Barbara's Day, the anniversary of Dr. Baeyer's first successful synthesis of the drug, is not clear. But the discovery's aftermath is well recorded in the pages of medical history.

By 1912 phenobarbital was being widely marketed as a potent sleeping aid, and dozens of other barbiturates with varying degrees of effectiveness were being developed.

While the precise way barbiturates work is unclear—they appear to interfere with nerve impulses within the brain—the results of their use are well documented and directly related to the dosages. Small doses have a sedative effect; they "calm the nerves." Somewhat larger doses can make you fall asleep.

Overdoses can lead to coma and death.

While tolerance to barbiturates builds with repeated usage, and increasingly larger doses are required to attain a sedative effect, the amount needed to cause death remains about the same. Thus for frequent users there remains a smaller and smaller margin of safety between an effective dose and a deadly dose. For this reason most physicians today urge their patients to periodically stop using barbiturates altogether for several days. These "therapeutic holidays" permit the body to eliminate most traces of the drugs and allow users on long-term drug therapy programs to return to lower doses.

Some barbiturates—phenobarbital, secobarbital, and amobarbital—are listed among the country's top 20 abused drugs.

Barbiturates are classed according to the speed with which they take effect, and the overall length of their action: ultra-short-acting, short-acting, intermediate-acting, and long-acting.

Short- and intermediate-acting barbiturates produce an effect similar to being drunk, what doctors and researchers call "disinhibition euphoria," during which normal inhibitions are suppressed. It is this euphoria which makes short- and intermediate-acting barbiturates attractive to people determined to abuse them.

Some heavy barbiturate users also insist they become sexually aroused when taking the drugs, but there is no independent evidence proving that these drugs enhance sexuality.

Long-acting barbiturates are seldom abused because it takes too long for their effects to be felt. However, regular use of any barbiturate can result in a buildup of tolerance, which may lead to psychological and/or physical dependence.

All barbiturates, depending on the dosage, can cause mood changes. They reduce anxiety and suppress feelings of guilt, while appearing to increase energy and self-confidence.

Barbiturates taken in small amounts do little to kill pain, and in some people may increase sensitivity to pain. At high doses, especially in combination with anticonvulsive medications, barbiturates are useful in controlling epileptic seizures.

Precautions

Do not take barbiturates together with alcohol, antihistamines, or other depressants. If you develop tolerance to one barbiturate, or to alcohol, you will be tolerant to all barbiturates and many other sedatives.

Barbiturates will slow you down both physically and mentally, so you should be extremely careful driving, operating machinery, or performing any other task that requires concentration and alertness.

These drugs are neutralized in the liver and eliminated from the body through the kidneys, so if you have any liver or kidney disorder—such as a problem urinating—you should not take barbiturates without being carefully monitored by a doctor.

You should not take barbiturates if you know of any sensitivity to them, or have any reason to suspect you may be sensitive.

If you have previously been addicted to any sedatives, sleeping pills, or alcohol, you should avoid barbiturates. Avoid these drugs as well if you have any disease affecting the respiratory system, such as asthma, or if you have a history of blood disorders.

Interactions

The power of barbiturates to make you sleepy or calm you down will be increased when they are taken together with alcohol, antihistamines, or other tranquilizers. The combination of any one of the above, particularly alcohol, with barbiturates is dangerous and can be deadly.

If you take barbiturates at the same time you are using anticoagulants (blood-thinning agents), muscle relaxants, or pain killers, the effect of the barbiturates and the other drugs will be lessened.

Common Side Effects

Drowsiness; lethargy; skin rash; and generally mild allergic reactions like running nose, watering eyes, and scratchy throat.

Serious Adverse Effects

Anemia; yellowing of the skin and eyes; dizziness; hangover; nausea; vomiting; diarrhea; fever; liver damage; nightmares; hallucinations; paradoxical excitement; and coma.

Dependence and Addiction

When taken in limited amounts—say, small daily doses for three months—barbiturates generally do not cause physical dependence, even though tolerance develops and psychological dependence can occur. Larger doses, however, can cause physical dependence much sooner. Five to ten times the normal dose of barbiturates—about 500 to 1000 mg. per day—will rapidly result in psychological and physical dependence.

Among a significant percentage of the population, even very small doses of barbiturates taken for only a few days can lead to withdrawal symptoms when the drugs are stopped. Among such individuals—usually those with a personal or family history of drug or alcohol dependence—tolerance to barbiturates develops quickly, and rapid dosage increases are necessary to achieve the same effect as the first doses while avoiding withdrawal symptoms.

Once a barbiturate habit has developed, the drugs can cause chronic suppression of the REM (rapid eye movement) phase of sleep. In recent years researchers have begun to study in detail such questions as why people sleep, how much sleep is needed, and why some individuals appear to sleep more restfully than others during, say, an eight-hour period. They learned that for most people, sleep is divided into several stages. During one of them, brain activity is minimal and there are virtually no dreams. During another, sleep is very light and close to wakefulness. During the REM phase of sleep dreams are frequent, and the eyes move back and forth as though watching a movie. This is the sleep phase during which most people appear to gain the greatest amount of rest. In tests during which REM sleep has continually been disturbed (the people were wakened whenever their eye movement showed they were in REM sleep), the subjects almost always felt tired the next morning and said later they had slept poorly.

Symptoms of dependence or addiction to barbiturates are much like the symptoms of chronic alcoholism: unsteady gait; slurred speech; confusion; poor judgment; irritability; insomnia; and poor sleep. Other symptoms include a compulsive need to take increasingly higher doses of barbiturates despite knowing the consequences, and a need to continue using the drugs to avoid the pain of withdrawal.

Withdrawal Symptoms

It is vital that barbiturate withdrawal symptoms be spotted

Adapin **25 mg** p. 259	**Adapin** **75 mg** p. 259	**Aventyl HCL** **25 mg** p. 261	**Carbrital** p. 161
Compazine Span. **10 mg** p. 247	**Compazine Span.** **15 mg** p. 247	**Dalmane** **15 mg** p. 195	**Dalmane** **30 mg** p. 195
Darvon **Compound** p. 231	**Darvon** **Compound-65** p. 231	**Dexedrine** **Spansules** p. 135	**Dexedrine Span.** **15 mg** p. 135
Fastin **30 mg** p. 128	**Fiorinal** **w/Cod. # 3** p. 220	**Librium** **5 mg** p. 192	**Librium** **10 mg** p. 192
Meprospan **200 mg** p. 203	**Meprospan** **400 mg** p. 203	**Nembutal Sodium** **50 mg** p. 156	**Pamelor** **25 mg** p. 261

A

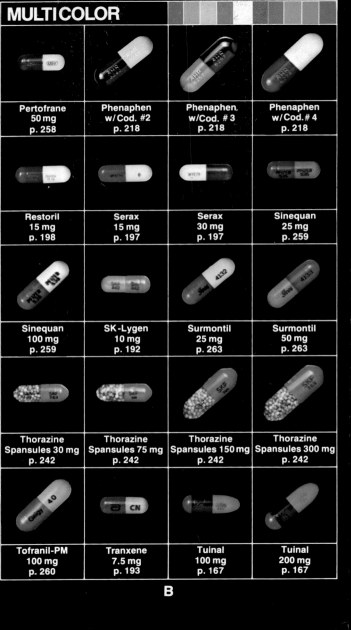

MULTICOLOR

Pertofrane 50 mg p. 258	**Phenaphen** w/Cod. #2 p. 218	**Phenaphen** w/Cod. # 3 p. 218	**Phenaphen** w/Cod. # 4 p. 218
Restoril 15 mg p. 198	**Serax** 15 mg p. 197	**Serax** 30 mg p. 197	**Sinequan** 25 mg p. 259
Sinequan 100 mg p. 259	**SK-Lygen** 10 mg p. 192	**Surmontil** 25 mg p. 263	**Surmontil** 50 mg p. 263
Thorazine Spansules 30 mg p. 242	**Thorazine** Spansules 75 mg p. 242	**Thorazine** Spansules 150 mg p. 242	**Thorazine** Spansules 300 mg p. 242
Tofranil-PM 100 mg p. 260	**Tranxene** 7.5 mg p. 193	**Tuinal** 100 mg p. 167	**Tuinal** 200 mg p. 167

B

MULTICOLOR

Vistaril 25 mg p. 206	Vistaril 50 mg p. 206		

WHITE/GRAY

A.P.C. w/Cod. # 3 p. 219	A.S.A. w/Cod. # 2 p. 219	Ativan 1 mg p. 196	Ativan 2 mg p. 196
Biphetamine 12.5 mg p. 132	Biphetamine 20 mg p. 132	Codeine Sulfate 30 mg p. 216	Cylert 18.75 mg p. 140
Demerol 50 mg p. 225	Desoxyn 5 mg p. 136	Doriden 500 mg p. 175	

C

WHITE/GRAY

Equanil 200 mg p. 203	Equanil 400 mg p. 203	Haldol .5 mg p. 244
Levo-Dromoran 2 mg p. 224	Mebaral 100 mg p. 155	Mellaril 50 mg p. 248
Meprobamate 400 mg p. 203	Miltown 400 mg p. 203	Phenobarbital 16 mg p. 157 / Phenobarbital 65 mg p. 157
Quaalude p. 178	Ritalin 10 mg p. 137	SK-Amitriptyline 10 mg p. 257
SK-65 p. 231	Tranxene 3.75 mg p. 193 / Tranxene 15 mg p. 193	Trilafon 2 mg p. 246

D

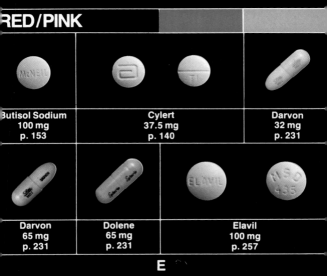

WHITE/GRAY

Trilafon 4 mg p. 246	Trilafon Repetabs 8 mg p. 246	Tylenol w/Codeine #2 p. 218	
Tylenol w/Codeine #3 p. 218		Valium 2 mg p. 194	Xanax 0.25 mg p. 192

RED/PINK

Butisol Sodium 100 mg p. 153	Cylert 37.5 mg p. 140		Darvon 32 mg p. 231
Darvon 65 mg p. 231	Dolene 65 mg p. 231	Elavil 100 mg p. 257	

E

RED/PINK

Haldol 2 mg p. 244	**Noctec** 500 mg p. 169	**Pertofrane** 25 mg p. 258	**Placidyl** 500 mg p. 172
Seconal Sodium 100 mg p. 158	**Sinequan** 10 mg p. 259	**Sinequan** 50 mg p. 259	**SK-Lygen** 5 mg p. 192

YELLOW

Atarax 50 mg p. 206	**Compazine** 5 mg p. 247	**Compazine** 10 mg. p. 247	**Elavil** 25 mg p. 257
Endep 75 mg p. 257	**Haldol** 1 mg p. 244	**Ionamin** 30 mg p. 128	**Mellaril** 10 mg p. 248

F

Mellaril 100 mg p. 248	**Nembutal Sodium** 100 mg p. 156	**Norpramin** 25 mg p. 258
Percodan p. 230	**Permitil** 1 mg p. 243	**Prochlorperazine** 5 mg p. 247	**Prochlorperazine** 10 mg p. 247
Prolixin 2.5 mg p. 243	**Ritalin** 5 mg p. 137	**Ritalin** 20 mg p. 137
SK-Amitriptyline 50 mg p. 257	**Sparine** 25 mg p. 248	**Valium** 5 mg p. 194	**Vivactil** 10 mg p. 262

BLUE/PURPLE

Amytal Sodium 200 mg p. 152	**Asendin** 100 mg p. 257	**Butisol Sodium** 15 mg p. 153	**Elavil** 10 mg p. 257
Lotusate 120 mg p. 159	**Percodan Demi** p. 230	**SK-Pramine** 25 mg p. 260	**SK-Pramine** 50 mg p. 260
Stelazine 1 mg p. 249	**Stelazine** 2 mg p. 249	**Stelazine** 5 mg p. 249	**Stelazine** 10 mg p. 249
Tranxene 3.75 mg p. 193	**Valium** 10 mg p. 194	**Vesprin** 10 mg p. 250	**Xanax** 1 mg p. 192

H

ORANGE

Adapin 10 mg p. 259	**Atarax** 10 mg p. 206	**Butisol Sodium** 50 mg p. 153	**Desoxyn** 10 mg p. 136
Dexedrine 5 mg p. 135	**Dilaudid** 2 mg p. 224	**Elavil** 75 mg p. 257	
Empracet w/Cod. # 3 p. 218	**Endep** 25 mg p. 257	**Endep** 50 mg p. 257	**Paxipam** 20 mg p. 196
Seconal Sodium 50 mg p. 158	**Sparine** 50 mg p. 248	**Talwin** 50 mg p. 210	**Thorazine** 10 mg p. 242
Thorazine 50 mg p. 242	**Thorazine** 100 mg p. 242	**Vivactil** 5 mg p. 262	**Xanax** 0.5 mg p. 192

I

GREEN

Butisol Sodium **30 mg** p. 153	**Centrax** **5 mg** p. 198	**Haldol** **5 mg** p. 244
Haldol **10 mg** p. 244	**Libritabs** **5 mg** p. 192	**Luminal** p. 157	**Norpramin** **50 mg** p. 258
Prolixin **5 mg** p. 243	**SK-Amitriptyline** **25 mg** p. 257	**SK-Chloral** **Hydrate 500 mg** p. 169	**Tybatran** **350 mg** p. 204
Wygesic p. 231		

J

BROWN

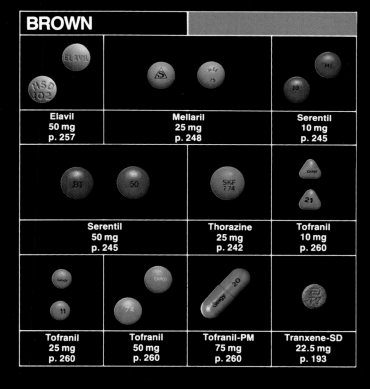

Elavil 50 mg p. 257	Mellaril 25 mg p. 248	Serentil 10 mg p. 245
Serentil 50 mg p. 245	Thorazine 25 mg p. 242	Tofranil 10 mg p. 260
Tofranil 25 mg p. 260	Tofranil 50 mg p. 260	Tofranil-PM 75 mg p. 260	Tranxene-SD 22.5 mg p. 193

K

LOOKALIKES

Lookalike #1 | **Lookalike #2** | **Lookalike #3** | **Lookalike #4**

Lookalike #5 | **Lookalike #6** | **Lookalike #7** | **Lookalike #8**

Lookalike #9 | **Lookalike #10** | **Lookalike #11** | **Lookalike #12**

Lookalike #13 | **Lookalike #14** | **Lookalike #15** | **Lookalike #16**

Lookalike #17 | **Lookalike #18** | **Lookalike #19** | **Lookalike #20**

L

LOOKALIKES

Lookalike #21	Lookalike #22	Lookalike #23	Lookalike #24
Lookalike #25	Lookalike #26	Lookalike #27	Lookalike #28
Lookalike #29	Lookalike #30	Lookalike #31	Lookalike #32
Lookalike #33	Lookalike #34	Lookalike #35	Lookalike #36

The products pictured on plates L-M are the lookalike pills. The pills on plates N-P are lookalike pills on top and their prescription counterparts on the bottom. Plate N is magnified 5 times normal size, plates O-P are magnified 2.3 times normal size.

M

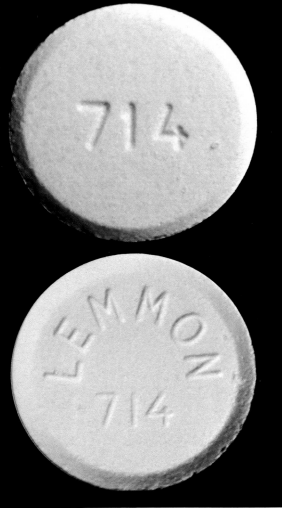

Lookalike #1
Quaalude
p. 178

N

LOOKALIKES

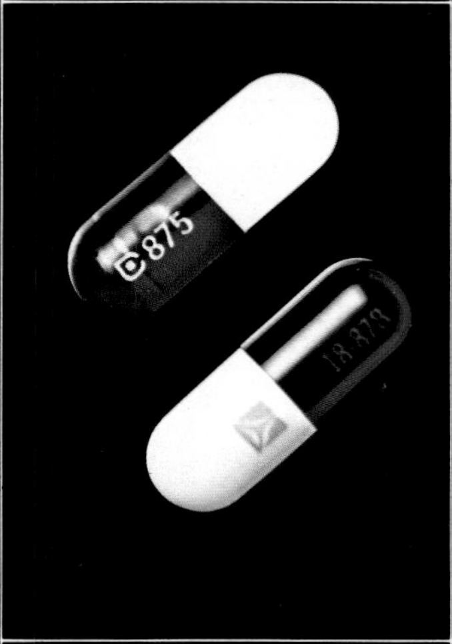

Lookalike #8
Biphetamine 12.5 mg
p. 132

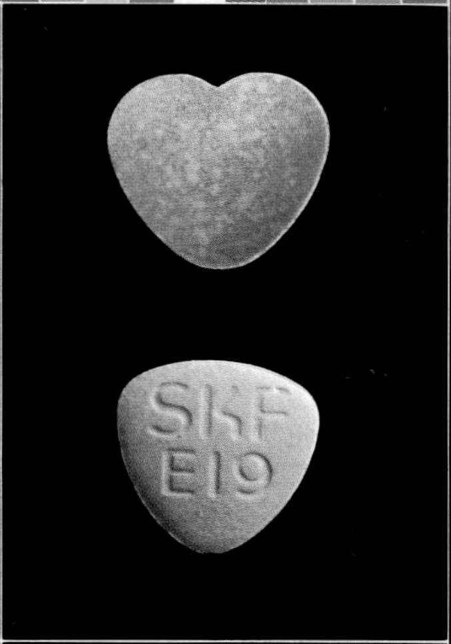

Lookalike #11
Dexedrine 5 mg
p. 135

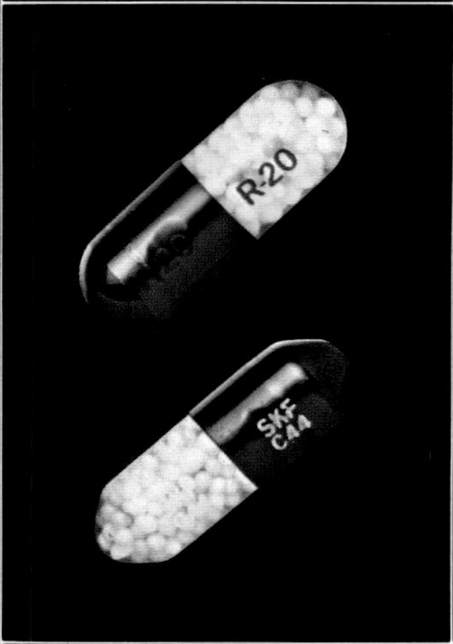

Lookalike #16
Compazine 10 mg
p. 247

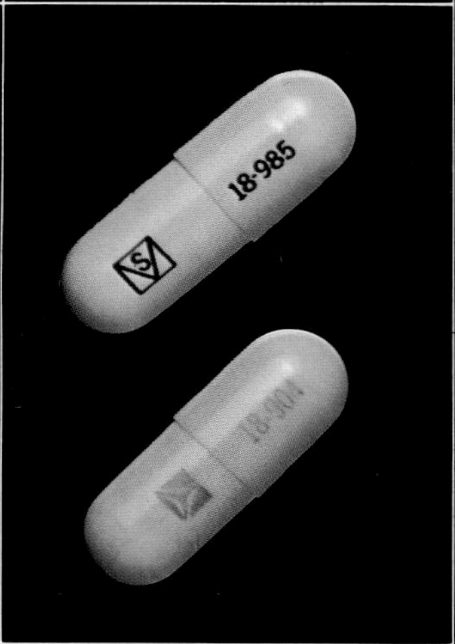

Lookalike #20
Ionamin 30 mg
p. 128

O

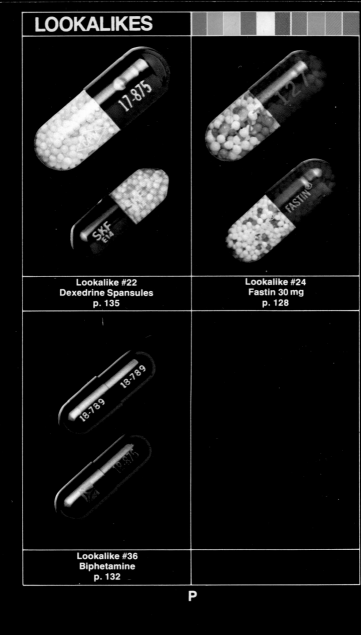

LOOKALIKES

Lookalike #22
Dexedrine Spansules
p. 135

Lookalike #24
Fastin 30 mg
p. 128

Lookalike #36
Biphetamine
p. 132

P

quickly; withdrawal can be severe, and can cause death if not managed by medical specialists.

Initial symptoms, which usually appear 8 to 12 hours after the last dose of barbiturates (they can take days to develop in some people), can include anxiety; twitching muscles; tremors of the hands and fingers; increasing weakness; dizziness; visual distortion; nausea; vomiting; severe insomnia; and vivid, disturbing dreams when sleep finally occurs.

More serious symptoms, which may occur within 16 hours and last five days or more after the most recent barbiturate dose, can include convulsions, disorientation to time, and delirium.

The symptoms of withdrawal gradually decline over a period of about two weeks.

Withdrawal Treatment

Because barbiturate withdrawal can threaten your health— and your life—so seriously, you should never stop taking them suddenly without medical supervision. If you are going to stop, you should consult a physician or visit a detoxification center, where a long-acting barbiturate can be substituted and the dosage gradually reduced until you are no longer addicted.

Overdose and Treatment

The effectiveness of barbiturates often wanes after a relatively short time (two weeks or less). As the body becomes accustomed to the drugs, a higher dosage is required to gain the same effect. The lethal dosage, however, remains about the same, so as usage grows, there is an increasingly fine line between an effective dosage and an overdose.

Nearly 5000 deaths, and thousands more emergency room visits, result each year from barbiturate overdoses, many of them occurring because barbiturates were taken along with alcohol, a particularly dangerous combination.

Symptoms of a moderate overdose are similar to those of an "overdose" of alcohol, when you drink too much.

A heavy overdose of barbiturates causes breathing trouble; a decrease in the size of the pupils of the eyes; lowered body temperature changing to fever within a few hours; fluid in the lungs; and eventually coma and the danger of death.

Anyone suspected of having taken an overdose of barbiturates must be taken to a hospital immediately. Always bring the pill bottle so the emergency room staff can quickly identify the medication and begin proper treatment without delay.

Medical treatment for barbiturate overdoses often includes forcing the victim to vomit (or pumping the stomach); having the victim swallow activated charcoal to absorb barbiturates remaining in the stomach; and taking other lifesaving measures that can be performed only by qualified medical personnel.

Usage in Pregnancy

Some studies have shown a relationship between barbiturates and birth defects. While not conclusive, they serve to warn pregnant women that they should carefully consider the need for any sedative against the potential harm to an unborn child.

Usage During Breast Feeding

Barbiturate traces are excreted in breast milk, and since the effect on infants has not been adequately studied, the safety of barbiturate use by nursing mothers has not been established.

Usage by the Elderly

Elderly people (those over 65) may become nervous or confused at times because of barbiturate usage, even at prescribed dosages. Since barbiturates cause the body temperature to drop, their use by the elderly should be closely supervised to avoid the common problem of hypothermia (reduced body temperature).

Usage by Children

Children taking barbiturates may become irritable, excitable, and aggressive, and may cry without reason. If a child becomes extremely excitable after taking barbiturates, he or she may be exhibiting a special sensitivity to the drug, and its use should be reconsidered.

BARBITURATES: ONSET AND DURATION

The chart shows how soon the drugs take effect: the solid lines show peak effect, while the broken lines show when most people are affected. (Traces of most barbiturates can be found in the body for days after their peaks.)

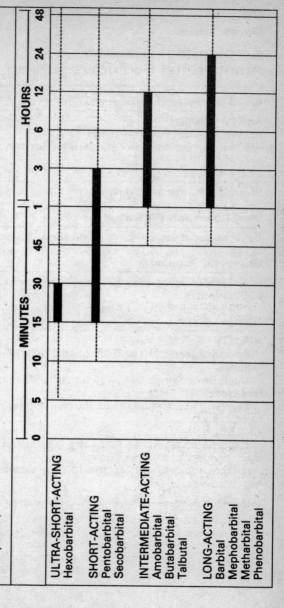

Generic Names

Amobarbital (Schedule II)
Amobarbital Sodium (Schedule II)

Brand Names (and Companies)

Amytal (Lilly)
Amytal Sodium Pulvules (Lilly)
Also sold generically as Amobarbital Sodium

Street Names

Blues; bluebirds; blue devils.

Most Commonly Prescribed for

Daytime sedative; sleeping medication; seizures.

Onset and Duration

Intermediate-acting (6 to 12 hours). Takes effect in about 45
to 60 minutes.

Dosage

ADULTS
   Anticonvulsant: 110 to 260 mg. total daily divided into 2 to
4 doses.
   Daytime sedative: 60 to 150 mg. total daily divided into 2
to 4 doses.
   Sleeping medication: 65 to 200 mg. at bedtime (rarely up
to 500 mg.).
CHILDREN
   Daytime sedative: 12 to 24 mg. per kg. of weight total
daily divided into 4 equal doses.
Available sizes: 15, 30, 50, and 100 mg. tablets; 65 and 200
mg. capsules.

Important: Precautions and warnings about this drug, pp 145–150

Generic Name

Barbital (Schedule IV)

Brand Name (and Company)

Barbital (Scrip)

Most Commonly Prescribed for

Sleeping medication; various types of anxiety; gastrointestinal ailments; hypertension.

Onset and Duration

Long-acting (12 to 24 hours). Takes effect in about 1 hour.

Dosage

ADULTS
   Daytime sedative: 110 to 390 mg. total daily divided into 2 to 3 doses.
   Hypertension, gastrointestinal ailments: Small doses depending on particular ailment and response to drug.
   Sleeping medication: 300 to 600 mg. at bedtime.

Important: Precautions and warnings about this drug, pp 145–150

Generic Name

Butabarbital Sodium (Schedule III)

Brand Names (and Companies)

Butal (Blaine)   Butisol Sodium (Wallace)
Butatran (Hauck)   Sarisol (Halsey)
Butazem (Zemmer)   Soduben (Arcum)
Buticaps (Wallace)
Also sold under generic name

Most Commonly Prescribed for

Daytime sedative; sleeping medication.

Onset and Duration

Intermediate-acting (6 to 12 hours). Takes effect in about 45 to 60 minutes.

Dosage

ADULTS
Daytime sedative: 45 to 120 mg. total daily divided into 3 to 4 doses.
Sleeping medication: 50 to 100 mg. at bedtime.
CHILDREN
Daytime sedative: 6 mg. per kg. of weight total daily divided into 3 doses.
Available sizes: 15, 16, 30, 32, 50, and 100 mg. tablets; 15, 30, 50, and 100 mg. capsules.

Important: Precautions and warnings about this drug, pp 145–150

Generic Name

Hexobarbital (Schedule III)

Brand Name (and Company)

Sombulex (Riker)

Most Commonly Prescribed for

Daytime sedative; sleeping medication.

Onset and Duration

Ultra-short-acting (15 minutes to 3 hours). Takes effect in about 5 to 15 minutes.

Dosage

ADULTS
Daytime sedative: 250 mg. repeated as needed every 2 to 3 hours.
Sleeping medication: 250 to 500 mg. at bedtime; when sleep has been interrupted, 250 mg. to restore sleep.
Available size: 250 mg. tablets.

Important: Precautions and warnings about this drug, pp 145–150

Generic Name
Mephobarbital (Schedule IV)

Brand Names (and Companies)

Mebaral (Breon)
Mephohab (Bowman)
Also sold under generic name

Most Commonly Prescribed for

Daytime sedative; anticonvulsant for the treatment of
epilepsy; alcohol withdrawal.

Onset and Duration

Long-acting (12 to 24 hours). Takes effect in about 1 hour.

Dosage

ADULTS
   Alcohol withdrawal: 600 mg. total daily divided into 3
doses.
   Daytime sedative: 96 to 400 mg. total daily divided into 3
to 4 doses.
   Epilepsy: 400 to 600 mg. total daily in divided doses.
CHILDREN
   Daytime sedative: 48 to 128 mg. total daily divided into 3
to 4 doses.
   Epilepsy: (5 and over) 96 to 256 mg. total daily divided
into 3 to 4 doses; (under 5) 48 to 128 mg. total daily
divided into 3 to 4 doses.
Available sizes: 32, 50, 100, and 200 mg. tablets.

Important: Precautions and warnings about this drug, pp 145–150

Generic Name
Metharbital (Schedule III)

Brand Name (and Company)

Gemonil (Abbott)

Most Commonly Prescribed for

Various types of seizures.

Onset and Duration

Long-acting (12 to 24 hours). Takes effect in about 1 hour.

Dosage

ADULTS
  Seizures: 100 to 300 mg. total daily divided into 1 to 3
doses gradually increased up to 800 mg. total daily.
CHILDREN
  Seizures: 5 to 15 mg. per kg. of weight total daily divided
into 3 doses gradually increased up to 300 mg. total daily
in divided doses.
Available size: 100 mg. tablets.

Important: Precautions and warnings about this drug, pp 145–150

Generic Names

Pentobarbital (Schedule II)
Pentobarbital Sodium (Schedule II)

Brand Names (and Companies)

Maso-Pent (Mason)
Nembutal Sodium (Abbott)
Night Caps (Bowman)
Penital (Kay)
Also sold generically as Pentobarbital Sodium

Street Names

Yellows; yellow jackets; nebbies; nemmies.

Most Commonly Prescribed for

Daytime sedative; sleeping medication.

Onset and Duration

Short-acting (3 to 6 hours). Takes effect in about 10 to 15
minutes.

Dosage

ADULTS
Daytime sedative: 40 to 160 mg. total daily divided into 2 to 4 doses.
Sleeping medication: 100 to 200 mg. at bedtime.
CHILDREN
Daytime sedative: 6 mg. per kg. of weight at bedtime.
Available sizes: 100 mg. tablets; 90 and 100 mg. prolonged-action tablets; 30, 50, and 100 mg. capsules.

Important: Precautions and warnings about this drug, pp 145–150

Generic Name

Phenobarbital (Schedule IV)

Brand Names (and Companies)

Bar (Scrip)   PBR/12 (Scott-Alison)
Barbipil (North American)   Pheno-Squar (Mallard)
Barbita (North American)   SK-Phenobarbital (SKF)
Eskabarb (SKF)   Solfoton (Poythress)
Henotal (Bowman)   Solu-barb (Fellows-Testagar)
Luminal Ovoids (Winthrop)   Stenal (Robins)
Also sold under generic name

Street Names

Purple hearts; barbs; candy; goofballs; peanuts.

Most Commonly Prescribed for

Daytime sedative; sleeping medication; convulsions; acute psychotic agitation.

Onset and Duration

Long-acting (12 to 24 hours). Takes effect in about 1 hour.

Dosage

ADULTS
Convulsions: 50 to 100 mg. total daily divided into 1 to 3 doses (usually 90 mg. total daily divided into 3 doses).

Daytime sedative: 30 to 64 mg. total daily in divided doses.

Sleeping medication: 100 to 300 mg. at bedtime.

CHILDREN

Convulsions: 32 to 150 mg. total daily divided into 2 to 3 doses.

Daytime sedative: 1 mg. per kg. of weight total daily in divided doses.

Sleeping medication: 3 to 6 mg. per kg. of weight at bedtime.

Available sizes: 8, 15, 16, 30, 32, 65, and 100 mg. tablets; 16, 65, and 100 mg. capsules; 65 mg. time-release capsules.

Important: Precautions and warnings about this drug, pp 145–150

Generic Names

Secobarbital (Schedule II)
Secobarbital Sodium (Schedule II)

Brand Names (and Companies)

Seconal Sodium Pulvules (Lilly)
Also sold generically as Secobarbital Sodium

Street Names

Reds; redbirds; red devils.

Most Commonly Prescribed for

Daytime sedative; sleeping medication.

Onset and Duration

Short-acting (3 to 6 hours). Takes effect in about 10 to 15 minutes.

Dosage

ADULTS

Daytime sedative: 30 to 50 mg. per dose, repeated as required.

Sleeping medication: 100 to 200 mg. at bedtime.

CHILDREN

Daytime sedative: 6 mg. per kg. of weight total daily divided into 3 doses.

Available sizes: 60 mg. tablets; 50 and 100 mg. capsules.

Important: Precautions and warnings about this drug, pp 145–150

Generic Name

Talbutal (Schedule III)

Brand Name (and Company)

Lotusate Caplets (Winthrop)

Street Name

Purple hearts.

Most Commonly Prescribed for

Sleeping medication.

Onset and Duration

Intermediate-acting (6 to 12 hours). Takes effect in about 45 to 60 minutes.

Dosage

ADULTS

Sleeping medication: 120 mg. at bedtime.

Available size: 120 mg. tablets.

Important: Precautions and warnings about this drug, pp. 145–150

BARBITURATE COMBINATIONS

These drugs combine two or more barbiturates, or barbiturates and pain killers, antihistamines, or other medications. Each component has a specific duration of action, and the combinations allow for optimal usage of each ingredient. This usually makes these drugs easier to take and more effective due to the differing rates of onset, duration, and metabolism in the body of the components.

Appropriate dosages should be determined by a physician only after careful study of a patient's condition. Because everyone will react differently to the combinations, no specific dosages are given with individual listings. However, the amount per capsule or tablet of each ingredient is provided so that readers will know the relative amounts contained in each drug.

Some of the ingredients listed in barbiturate combination pills are not described in detail under their own generic names since they are not available alone in tablet or capsule form, but only as elixirs or preparations made for injection.

The same general information applies to these drugs as to individual barbiturates; readers are advised to refer to the warnings above (pp. 145–150) before using barbiturate combination drugs.

Brand Name (and Company)

Butatrax (Sutliff & Case) (Schedule II)

Ingredients

Amobarbital. Intermediate-acting (6 to 12 hours). Takes effect in about 1 hour. (20 mg.)

Butabarbital. Intermediate-acting (6 to 12 hours). Takes effect in about 45 to 60 minutes. (30 mg.)

Most Commonly Prescribed for

Daytime sedative; sleeping medication.
Available size: 50 mg. capsules.

Important: Precautions and warnings about this drug, pp 145–150

Brand Name (and Company)

Butseco (Bowman) (Schedule II)

Ingredients

Phenobarbital. Long-acting (12 to 24 hours). Takes effect in about 1 hour. (16 mg.)

Butabarbital Sodium. Intermediate-acting (6 to 12 hours). Takes effect in about 45 to 60 minutes. (16 mg.)

Secobarbital Sodium. Short-acting (3 to 6 hours). Takes effect in about 10 to 15 minutes. (16 mg.)

Most Commonly Prescribed for

Daytime sedative; sleeping medication.
Available size: 48 mg. tablets.

Important: Precautions and warnings about this drug, pp 145–150

Brand Name (and Company)

Carbrital Kapseals (Parke-Davis) (Schedule III)

Ingredients

Pentobarbital Sodium. Short-acting (3 to 6 hours). Takes effect in about 10 to 15 minutes. (97.5 mg.)

Carbromal. Short-acting (3 to 6 hours). Takes effect in about 10 to 15 minutes. (260 mg.)

Most Commonly Prescribed for

Daytime sedative; sleeping medication.

General Information

Carbrital Kapseals have been placed on the Food and Drug Administration's list of drugs considered "less than effective." Available size: 357.5 mg. capsules.

Important: Precautions and warnings about this drug, pp 145–150

Brand Name (and Company)

Ethobral (Wyeth) (Schedule II)

Ingredients

Phenobarbital. Long-acting (12 to 24 hours). Takes effect in about 1 hour. (50 mg.)

Butabarbital Sodium. Intermediate-acting (6 to 12 hours). Takes effect in about 45 to 60 minutes. (30 mg.)

Secobarbital Sodium. Short-acting (3 to 6 hours). Takes effect in about 10 to 15 minutes. (50 mg.)

Most Commonly Prescribed for

Daytime sedative; sleeping medication.
Available size: 130 mg. capsules.

Important: Precautions and warnings about this drug, pp 145–150

Brand Name (and Company)

Hyptran (Wallace) (Schedule III)

Ingredients

Secobarbital. Short-acting (3 to 6 hours). Takes effect in about 10 to 15 minutes. (60 mg.)

Phenyltoloxamine Dihydrogen Citrate (antihistamine). (100 mg.)

Most Commonly Prescribed for

Daytime sedative; sleeping medication.
Available size: 160 mg. tablets.

Important: Precautions and warnings about this drug, pp 145–150

Brand Name (and Company)

Lull (Foy) (Schedule III)

Ingredients

Phenobarbital Sodium. Long-acting (12 to 24 hours). Takes effect in about 1 hour. (16 mg.)

Butabarbital Sodium. Intermediate-acting (6 to 12 hours). Takes effect in about 45 to 60 minutes. (16 mg.)

Most Commonly Prescribed for

Daytime sedative; sleeping medication.
Available size: 32 mg. tablets.

Important: Precautions and warnings about this drug, pp 145–150

Brand Name (and Company)

Nidar (Armour) (Schedule II)

Ingredients

Phenobarbital Sodium. Long-acting (12 to 24 hours). Takes effect in about 1 hour. (7.5 mg.)

Butabarbital Sodium. Intermediate-acting (6 to 12 hours). Takes effect in about 45 to 60 minutes. (7.5 mg.)

Secobarbital Sodium. Short-acting (3 to 6 hours). Takes effect in about 10 to 15 minutes. (25 mg.)

Pentobarbital Sodium. Short-acting (3 to 6 hours). Takes effect in about 10 to 15 minutes. (25 mg.)

Most Commonly Prescribed for

Daytime sedative; sleeping medication.
Available size: 65 mg. tablets.

Important: Precautions and warnings about this drug, pp 145–150

Brand Name (and Company)

Penotal (Coastal) (Schedule II)

Ingredients

Phenobarbital Sodium. Long-acting (12 to 24 hours). Takes effect in about 1 hour. (24 mg.)

Pentobarbital Sodium. Short-acting (3 to 6 hours). Takes effect in about 10 to 15 minutes. (24 mg.)

Most Commonly Prescribed for

Daytime sedative; sleeping medication.
Available size: 48 mg. capsules.

Important: Precautions and warnings about this drug, pp 145–150

Brand Name (and Company)

Plexonal (Sandoz) (Schedule III)

Ingredients

Barbital Sodium. Long-acting (12 to 24 hours). Takes effect in about 1 hour. (45 mg.)

Phenobarbital Sodium. Long-acting (12 to 24 hours). Takes effect in about 1 hour. (15 mg.)

Butalbital Sodium. Short-acting (1 to 6 hours). Takes effect in about 10 to 15 minutes. (25 mg.)

Dihydroergotamine Mesylate (pain killer). (0.16 mg.)

Scopolamine HBr (antispasmodic). (0.08 mg.)

Most Commonly Prescribed for

Daytime sedative; sleeping medication.
Available size: 85.24 mg. tablets.

Important: Precautions and warnings about this drug, pp 145–150

Brand Name (and Company)

Quan III (Mallard) (Schedule III)

Ingredients

Phenobarbital. Long-acting (12 to 24 hours). Takes effect in about 1 hour. (25 mg.)

Butabarbital. Intermediate-acting (6 to 12 hours). Takes effect in about 45 to 60 minutes. (50 mg.)

Aprobarbital. Intermediate-acting (6 to 12 hours). Takes effect in about 45 to 60 minutes. (25 mg.)

Most Commonly Prescribed for

Daytime sedative; sleeping medication.
Available size: 100 mg. tablets.

Important: Precautions and warnings about this drug, pp 145–150

Brand Name (and Company)

S.B.P. (Lemmon) (Schedule II)

Ingredients

Phenobarbital. Long-acting (12 to 24 hours). Takes effect in about 1 hour. (15 mg.)

Butabarbital Sodium. Intermediate-acting (6 to 12 hours). Takes effect in about 45 to 60 minutes. (30 mg.)

Secobarbital sodium. Short-acting (3 to 6 hours). Takes effect in about 10 to 15 minutes. (50 mg.)

Most Commonly Prescribed for

Daytime sedative; sleeping medication.
Available size: 95 mg. tablets.

Important: Precautions and warnings about this drug, pp 145–150

Brand Name (and Company)

Secanap (Zemmer) (Schedule II)

Ingredients

Phenobarbital. Long-acting (12 to 24 hours). Takes effect in about 1 hour. (30 mg.)

Secobarbital Sodium. Short-acting (3 to 6 hours). Takes effect in about 10 to 15 minutes. (30 mg.)

Pentobarbital Sodium. Short-acting (3 to 6 hours). Takes effect in about 10 to 15 minutes. (30 mg.)

Most Commonly Prescribed for

Daytime sedative; sleeping medication.
Available size: 90 mg. tablets.

Important: Precautions and warnings about this drug, pp 145–150

Brand Name (and Company)

Secophen (Mallard) (Schedule II)

Ingredients

Phenobarbital. Long-acting (12 to 24 hours). Takes effect in about 1 hour. (16 mg.)

Secobarbital Sodium. Short-acting (3 to 6 hours). Takes effect in about 10 to 15 minutes. (48 mg.)

Most Commonly Prescribed for

Daytime sedative; sleeping medication.
Available size: 64 mg. tablets.

Important: Precautions and warnings about this drug, pp 145–150

Brand Name (and Company)

Tri-Barbs (Lannett) (Schedule II)

Ingredients

Phenobarbital. Long-acting (12 to 24 hours). Takes effect in about 1 hour. (32 mg.)

Butabarbital Sodium. Intermediate-acting (6 to 12 hours). Takes effect in about 45 to 60 minutes. (32 mg.)

Secobarbital Sodium. Short-acting (3 to 6 hours). Takes effect in about 10 to 15 minutes. (32 mg.)

Most Commonly Prescribed for

Daytime sedative; sleeping medication.
Available size: 96 mg. capsules.

Important: Precautions and warnings about this drug, pp 145–150

Brand Name (and Company)

Tuinal Pulvules (Lilly) (Schedule II)

Ingredients

Amobarbital Sodium. Intermediate-acting (6 to 12 hours). Takes effect in about 45 to 60 minutes. (25, 50, or 100 mg.)

Secobarbital Sodium. Short-acting (3 to 6 hours). Takes effect in about 10 to 15 minutes. (25, 50, or 100 mg.)

Street Names

Christmas trees; rainbows; tooies; trees; double trouble.

Most Commonly Prescribed for

Daytime sedative; sleeping medication.
Available sizes: 50, 100, and 200 mg. capsules.

Important: Precautions and warnings about this drug, pp 145–150

Brand Name (and Company)

Twinbarbital #2 (Rugby) (Schedule II)

Ingredients

Amobarbital Sodium. Intermediate-acting (6 to 12 hours). Takes effect in about 45 to 60 minutes. (100 mg.)

Secobarbital Sodium. Short-acting (3 to 6 hours). Takes effect in about 10 to 15 minutes. (100 mg.)

Most Commonly Prescribed for

Daytime sedative; sleeping medication.
Available size: 200 mg. capsules.

Important: Precautions and warnings about this drug, pp 145–150

BARBITURATELIKE SEDATIVES

These drugs, while not chemically related to barbiturates, work similarly. They exert their effects in the central nervous system and are subject to widespread abuse.

Like barbiturates, they can cause physical and psychological dependence. Withdrawal can be extremely dangerous—even deadly—without the support of qualified medical personnel.

When sold illegally on the streets of large cities, or in school hallways across the country, they are often referred to by the same street names as barbiturates ("barbs," "candy," etc.) or by their own street names.

Generic Name

Chloral Hydrate (Schedule IV)

Brand Names (and Companies)

Cohidrate (Coastal)
HS-Need (Hanlon)
Noctec (Squibb)
Oradrate (Coast)
SK-Chloral Hydrate (SKF)
Also sold under generic name

Street Names

When combined with alcohol: Mickey; Peter; Mickey Finn; knockout drops.

Most Commonly Prescribed for

Daytime sedative; sleeping medication.

General Information

Chloral hydrate was romanticized in old movies as a Mickey Finn, or knockout drops, because when put into alcohol it can be very effective in causing sleep within an hour. Such films failed to indicate, however, that combining the drug with alcohol can often be deadly.

Precautions

Do not take this drug together with alcohol or other sedatives.

Do not take chloral hydrate if you have any liver or kidney diseases, severe heart trouble, or stomach problems, or if you suspect you are sensitive or allergic to this or similar drugs. Also, do not take this drug if you suffer from marked liver or kidney impairment, severe cardiac disease, or gastritis. Because this drug can cause drowsiness, you should be careful if you are driving, operating potentially dangerous machinery, or performing some other task that requires concentration and alertness.

Interactions

Taking chloral hydrate with blood-thinning drugs may require a dosage change of the latter. Chloral hydrate is a potent depressant, so do not drink alcohol or take any other sedative drugs while using this medication.

Common Side Effects

Lightheaded feeling; general weakness.

Serious Adverse Effects

Headache; hangover; hallucinations; stomach upset; nausea; vomiting; difficulty in walking; bad taste in the mouth; feeling of excitement; itching; dizziness; nightmares; and changes in the composition of the blood.

Dependence and Addiction

Tolerance to this drug develops rapidly, and dependence on chloral hydrate may become apparent as early as the second week of continued use. Some habitual users, who exhibit symptoms similar to alcoholism, take as much as 12 grams nightly.

Withdrawal Symptoms

Tremors; anxiety; hallucinations; and delirium.

Withdrawal Treatment

Treatment of chloral hydrate withdrawal usually involves a gradual reduction of the drug under close medical supervision.

Overdose Symptoms and Treatment

Symptoms of an overdose may include low body temperature; pinpoint pupils; irregular breathing; vomiting; and coma.

Anyone suspected of having taken an overdose of chloral hydrate must be taken to a hospital immediately. Always bring the pill bottle so the emergency room staff can quickly identify the medication and begin proper treatment, which usually includes emptying the stomach and performing other lifesaving measures.

Usage in Pregnancy

Safety for use during pregnancy has not been established.

Usage During Breast Feeding

Because chloral hydrate appears in breast milk, it is not recommended for use by nursing mothers.

Usage by the Elderly

The lowest effective dosage may be used.

Usage by Children

The lowest effective dosage may be used.

Onset and Duration

Intermediate-acting (6 to 12 hours). Takes effect in about 45 to 60 minutes.

Dosage

ADULTS

Daytime sedative: 750 mg. total daily divided into 3 doses (rarely up to 2000 mg.)

Sleeping medication: 500 to 1000 mg. before bedtime.

CHILDREN

Daytime sedative: 25 mg. per kg. of weight total daily divided into 3 doses.

Sleeping medication: 50 mg. per kg. of weight at bedtime up to a maximum of 1000 mg.

Available sizes: 250 and 500 mg. capsules.

Generic Name

Ethchlorvynol (Schedule IV)

Brand Name (and Company)

Placidyl (Abbott)

Most Commonly Prescribed for

Sleeping medication.

Precautions

Do not use Placidyl together with alcohol or other depressants.

Because Placidyl may cause drowsiness, you should be careful if you are driving, operating potentially dangerous machinery, or performing some other task that requires concentration and alertness.

If you have reason to suspect you are allergic to this drug, or if you experience skin rash or porphyria, you should not take Placidyl.

Do not take this drug for prolonged periods, since tolerance builds up in about 10 days and the drug's effectiveness beyond that time is doubtful.

The 750 mg. capsules contain tartrazine, which can cause allergic reactions in those sensitive to aspirin.

Interactions

The combination of Placidyl and amitriptyline (a tricyclic antidepressant) can make you become delirious.

Do not take this drug with alcohol, other depressants, or antihistamines.

Common Side Effects

Dizziness; blurred vision; and giddiness. The giddy feeling can be reduced by taking Placidyl shortly after the evening meal.

Serious Adverse Effects

Skin rash; nausea; morning-after hangover; facial numbness; nightmares; muscular weakness; vomiting; low blood pressure; incoordination; loss of memory; tremors; confusion; slurred speech; exaggeration of reflexes; double vision; and generalized muscle weakness.

Dependence and Addiction

When taken in sufficiently large doses over a period of several weeks, users will develop tolerance to this drug, and physical and psychological dependence can result.

Withdrawal Symptoms

Severe withdrawal symptoms similar to those seen during barbiturate and alcohol withdrawal occur following abrupt discontinuance of Placidyl. Symptoms may appear up to nine days after the last dose, and may include convulsions; delirium; schizoid reaction; perceptual distortions; memory loss; ataxia; insomnia; slurring of speech; unusual anxiety; irritability; agitation; tremors; loss of appetite (anorexia); nausea; vomiting; weakness; dizziness; sweating; muscle twitching; and weight loss.

Withdrawal Treatment

Because withdrawal from Placidyl can threaten your life, treatment should be handled only by qualified medical personnel. Treatment usually involves providing the same dosage of the drug as was being used previously, then gradually reducing the dosage. In some cases, a barbiturate is substituted before the dosage reduction. If psychotic symptoms occur during withdrawal, a phenothiazine drug is sometimes provided.

Overdose Symptoms and Treatment

Large overdoses can be fatal, and Placidyl is frequently

used in suicide attempts. Symptoms of severe overdose are coma; lowered body temperature followed by fever; absence of normal pain responses; and shallow breathing.

Anyone suspected of having taken an overdose of Placidyl must be taken to a hospital emergency room immediately. Always bring the pill bottle so the emergency room staff can quickly identify the medication and begin proper treatment, which may include pumping the stomach and other lifesaving measures.

Usage in Pregnancy

Not recommended.

Usage During Breast Feeding

Safety for use by nursing mothers has not been established.

Usage by the Elderly

The smallest effective dosage may be used.

Usage by Children

Not recommended for children under 15.

Onset and Duration

Intermediate-acting (6 to 12 hours). Takes effect in about 45 to 60 minutes.

Dosage

ADULTS
   Insomnia: 500 to 1000 mg. at bedtime.
Available sizes: 100, 200, 500, and 750 mg. capsules.

Generic Name

Glutethimide (Schedule III)

Brand Names (and Companies)

Doriden (USV)
Dormtabs (Spencer-Mead)
Rolathimide (Robinson)
Also sold under generic name

Street Names

Loads; setups (when combined with codeine).

Most Commonly Prescribed for

Sleeping medication.

General Information

Glutethimide in recent years has become increasingly popular among drug users when mixed with codeine. The two drugs, together known as "loads," are exceptionally dangerous, and have been responsible for several hundred overdose deaths across the country since 1980.

Dangerous enough when used individually, glutethimide and codeine used together offer users a "high" similar to that of heroin, which is not legal for any purpose in America. And overdose symptoms of the "loads" combination cannot be easily reversed by drugs usually used to minimize the effects of codeine.

The practice of using the two drugs to replace heroin appears to have begun on the west coast; it quickly spread to the northeast. Most often the two ingredients are stolen from drug supply facilities, prescribed by unscrupulous doctors, or sold illegally by pharmacists. On the street, "loads" are bought for somewhat less than half the price of heroin, for a dose providing the same effect.

Precautions

Do not use glutethimide together with alcohol or other depressants. This drug should not be used if you have any reason to suspect you are sensitive or allergic to it. Because glutethimide may cause dizziness and drowsiness, you should be careful if you are driving, operating potentially dangerous machinery, or performing some other task that requires concentration or alertness. Glutethimide is not recommended for prolonged use because tolerance builds rapidly, and its effectiveness beyond 7 days is doubtful.

Interactions

Do not take this drug together with alcohol, other sedatives, or antihistamines.

Doses of anticoagulant (blood-thinning) drugs may require adjustment because of the increased effects caused by glutethimide.

Common Side Effects

Skin rash; nausea; morning hangover; paradoxical excitation; and blurred vision.

Serious Adverse Effects

Changes in blood composition; vertigo; diarrhea; and generalized skin rash.

Dependence and Addiction

Physical and psychological addiction can result from prolonged use of this drug alone, or in combination with codeine.

Withdrawal Symptoms

Nausea; abdominal discomfort; tremors; convulsions; delirium; chills; numbness of extremities; and seizures.

Withdrawal Treatment

Glutethimide should be withdrawn gradually over a period of days or weeks under medical supervision.

Overdose Symptoms and Treatment

Large doses of glutethimide can be fatal, and the drug is frequently used in suicide attempts. Overdose symptoms can include coma; lowered body temperature followed by fever; absence of normal pain responses; and shallow breathing.

Anyone suspected of having taken an overdose of glutethimide must be taken to a hospital immediately. Always bring the pill bottle so the emergency room staff can quickly identify the medication and begin proper treatment without delay.

Treatment usually requires regular monitoring of vital signs; a continuous electrocardiogram to detect heart problems; maintenance of blood pressure; and, if absolutely essential, the use of pressor drugs.

People who use glutethimide for a long time may show signs of chronic overdosage: loss of memory; inability to concentrate; shakes; tremors; loss of reflexes; slurred speech; and a general sense of depression. Chronic overdosage is best treated by withdrawing the drug over a period of days or weeks.

Usage in Pregnancy

Not recommended.

Usage During Breast Feeding

Not recommended.

Usage by the Elderly

The lowest effective dosages may be used.

Usage by Children

Not recommended.

Onset and Duration

Intermediate-acting (6 to 12 hours). Takes effect in about 45 to 60 minutes.

Dosage

ADULTS
   250 to 500 mg. at bedtime.
Available sizes: 250 and 500 mg. tablets; 500 mg. capsules.

Generic Name

Methaqualone (Schedule II)

Brand Names (and Companies)

Mequin (Lemmon)   Quaalude (Lemmon)
Parest (Lemmon)   Sopor (Arnar-Stone)

Street Names

Ludes; quas; quads; soapers; sopes.

Most Commonly Prescribed for

Daytime sedative; sleeping medication.

General Information

Methaqualone's exact site of action is not known, although
it has sedative effects similar to those of barbiturates. The
so-called "sensual" effects that users claim to experience
indicate it may act at a different point in the central nervous system.

"Ludes" are among America's most controversial drugs.
They are number three on government lists of the 20 most
abused drugs, behind only heroin and diazepam (Valium).
In one recent year methaqualone was responsible for nearly
6000 emergency room visits and well over 100 overdose
deaths in this country.

Originally marketed in the early 1970s (by William H.
Rorer, Inc., which sold the brand name to Lemmon in
September 1978) as safe, effective, nonaddicting substi-
tutes for barbiturates, they are now considered to be one
of the most abused drugs still legally prescribed. Following
its original release, methaqualone quickly became the
nation's sixth best-selling sedative. It is now almost as
tightly controlled as heroin. Five states (Connecticut, Florida,
Georgia, Mississippi, and New Jersey) classify methaqualone as a Schedule I drug and have banned its distribution.
It is a widely distributed black market drug, manufactured
illegally in other countries and imported into the United
States.

One of the most severe problems associated with methaqualone abuse is that often the drug sold on the streets is a "counterfeit" pill. Illegal methaqualone powder is manufactured in Europe, then pressed into tablets in South America and smuggled into the U.S. for street sales. These pills are not manufactured carefully, and can contain toxic dose levels.

Methaqualone has often been prescribed by so-called stress clinics where people received expensive prescriptions for the drug, even though their physical conditions did not actually indicate a need for it.

Methaqualone has been linked to many overdose suicides and accidental deaths while driving.

Users of this drug claim that in addition to producing a euphoric and sensual state of relaxation, "ludes" also have aphrodisiacal properties. These effects, if they are more than imagination, are probably due to the drug's muscle relaxant qualities, which also can cause a lack of coordination.

Precautions

Do not take this drug together with alcohol or other sedatives.

Methaqualone is as dangerous as any barbiturate or other sedative. Those who are sensitive or allergic to any sedative should not use methaqualone, nor should anyone sensitive to methaqualone itself.

This drug is particularly dangerous when combined with alcohol, because the combination will greatly enhance the sedative effects of methaqualone. Most deaths associated with it are a result of just such a combination. Special precaution should be used when taking methaqualone and over-the-counter products containing alcohol.

Because methaqualone may cause drowsiness and slow down physical and mental reflexes, you should be extremely careful if you are driving, operating potentially dangerous machinery, or performing some other task that requires concentration and alertness.

Do not take this drug if you have any liver disease.

Interactions

Avoid combining methaqualone with alcohol; other sleeping medications; antihistamines; tranquilizers; and other depressants. Such combinations can lead to coma and death.

Common Side Effects

Headache; hangover; fatigue; nausea; dizziness; and skin rash.

Serious Adverse Effects

Tingling in the extremities; restlessness and anxiety; anemias; dry mouth; loss of appetite (anorexia); vomiting; diarrhea; stomach upset; sweating; and itching.

Dependence and Addiction

Tolerance, and both psychological and physical dependence, can develop from regular high-dose use of methaqualone. The potential for dependence is particularly great among people with a past personal or family history of alcoholism or drug addiction.

Symptoms of methaqualone addiction include irritability; sleeplessness; delirium tremens; mania; and convulsions.

Withdrawal Symptoms

Suddenly stopping the regular, long-term use of methaqualone can result in severe withdrawal symptoms including nausea; vomiting; nervousness; trembling; headache; anxiety; confusion; weakness; abdominal cramps; insomnia; nightmares; hallucinations; and convulsions.

Withdrawal Treatment

This drug must be gradually withdrawn to avoid the many serious withdrawal symptoms. Withdrawal should take place in a hospital setting.

Overdose Symptoms and Treatment

The most common symptoms of acute methaqualone overdose are convulsions; lowered body temperature followed by fever; absence of normal pain responses; shallow breathing; delirium; and coma.

Anyone suspected of having taken an overdose of methaqualone must be rushed to a hospital immediately. Always bring the pill bottle so emergency room staff can quickly identify the medication and begin proper treatment, which usually includes assuring an adequate oxygen supply and causing vomiting or pumping the victim's stomach. Stimulant drugs should never be used to try reversing the overdose symptoms.

People using methaqualone for long periods of time may also show signs of chronic overdose, including loss of memory; inability to concentrate; shakes; tremors; loss of reflexes; slurred speech; and a general sense of depression. Treatment includes gradual withdrawal of the drug and the substitution of a long-acting barbiturate such as phenobarbital, which is then gradually withdrawn.

Usage in Pregnancy

Not recommended.

Usage During Breast Feeding

Not recommended.

Usage by the Elderly

Small individualized doses may be used until the response is known.

Usage by Children

Not recommended.

Onset and Duration

Long-acting (12 to 24 hours). Takes effect in about 1 hour.

Dosage

ADULTS
Daytime sedative: 225 to 300 mg. total daily divided into 3 to 4 doses.
Sleeping medication: 150 to 300 mg. at bedtime.
Available sizes: 150 and 300 mg. tablets; 200 and 400 mg. capsules (containing methaqualone hydrochloride, equivalent in strength to 175 and 350 mg., respectively, of methaqualone).

Generic Name

Methyprylon (Schedule III)

Brand Name (and Company)

Noludar (Roche)

Most Commonly Prescribed for

Sleeping medication.

Precautions

Do not take Noludar together with alcohol, antihistamines, or other sedatives.

Avoid this drug if you suffer from porphyria.

Because Noludar may cause drowsiness, you should be careful if you are driving, operating potentially dangerous machinery, or performing some other task that requires concentration and alertness.

If you have reason to suspect you are allergic to this drug, perhaps due to previous experience with it, avoid using Noludar until the degree of your sensitivity has been determined by a physician.

Interactions

Antihistamines, alcohol, and other depressant drugs may increase the sedative effect of Noludar, and should be avoided.

Common Side Effects

Dizziness.

Serious Adverse Effects

Drowsiness the next morning; moderate stomach upset; headache; and skin rash.

Dependence and Addiction

When taken in large doses, over a period of several weeks, physical and psychological dependence on Noludar can develop.

Withdrawal Symptoms

Withdrawal symptoms similar to those seen during barbiturate withdrawal may follow abrupt discontinuance of Noludar, including convulsions; delirium; insomnia; slurring of speech; irritability; agitation; and tremors.

Withdrawal Treatment

Withdrawal from Noludar dependence should be handled by qualified medical personnel. Treatment usually involves maintaining the dosage of the drug, then gradually reducing it.

Overdose Symptoms and Treatment

Confusion; somnolence; constricted eye pupils; slow breathing; lowered blood pressure; and sometimes coma. Anyone suspected of having taken an overdose of Noludar must be taken to a hospital immediately. Always bring the pill bottle so the emergency room staff can quickly identify the medication and begin proper treatment without delay.

Treatment often involves pumping the victim's stomach, administering fluids intravenously, and giving drugs to raise blood pressure. Caffeine may be used to stimulate the victim. When convulsions occur during treatment of Noludar overdose, a barbiturate may be administered to control them.

Usage in Pregnancy

Not recommended.

Usage During Breast Feeding

Safety of use of this drug by nursing mothers has not been established.

Usage by the Elderly

The smallest effective dosage may be used.

Usage by Children

Not recommended for children under 12.

Onset and Duration

Long-acting (6 to 12 hours). Takes effect in about 30 to 60 minutes.

Dosage

ADULTS
   Insomnia: 200 to 400 mg. at bedtime.
CHILDREN (over 12)
   Insomnia: 50 to 200 mg. at bedtime.
Available sizes: 50 and 200 mg. tablets; 300 mg. capsules.

BENZODIAZEPINES

The most commonly prescribed group of sedatives is the benzodiazepines, which include such brand names as Valium and Librium.

Diazepam—the generic name for Valium—tops the federal government's list of the 20 most abused drugs in America, surpassing even heroin. With nearly 17,000 diazepam-caused emergency room visits reported during one recent year, compared with half as many related to heroin, diazepam demonstrates clearly the dangers of these drugs. Two other benzodiazepines, flurazepam (Dalmane) and chlordiazepoxide (Librium), are cited by the government on the same list for the high number of emergency room visits, and deaths, they cause.

The chemicals that later became these famous—and infamous—drugs were first developed in 1933, but for more than 20 years were considered too insignificant to warrant further study. In the mid-1950s, however, researchers administered chlordiazepoxide to several aggressive laboratory monkeys. They found that in small doses, less than the amounts required for putting the monkeys to sleep, the drug made the animals quite tame.

The Swiss-based multinational drug company Hoffmann-La Roche, learning of the surprising results on monkeys, began conducting human tests, and within a few years had started marketing chlordiazepoxide.

The firm called the drug Librium.

Librium was widely accepted by physicians and prescribed to patients. Researchers developed another benzodiazepine, diazepam, which was aggressively sold under the brand name Valium and has become the most widely prescribed benzodiazepine, and one of America's most popular drugs of all times.

Benzodiazepines have many important uses in medicine. They are prescribed as antianxiety agents, muscle relaxants, anticonvulsants, and sleeping pills, and are used to treat the symptoms of alcohol withdrawal.

Their tension-reducing properties have led them to be called "downs" by both patients receiving the drugs under prescription, and others selling or buying them illicitly. Americans consume more than 5,000,000,000 (five billion!)

legally purchased benzodiazepines annually, and countless millions more are bought on the streets, in schools, in offices, and elsewhere.

Some benzodiazepines are short-acting; after they exert their influence in the body, they are quickly excreted. Others are longer-lasting. All have about the same potential for abuse. Benzodiazepines alone rarely cause death; it is virtually impossible to kill yourself with an overdose. It has been said that the only way a research animal can die from benzodiazepines is by being crushed under a truckload of Valium pills.

But when the drugs are combined with alcohol the danger of overdose, death, or serious illness is substantially increased, and most of the benzodiazepine overdose cases that end up in hospital emergency rooms are alcohol combination cases. It is a tragedy that countless thousands of people deliberately take these drugs with alcohol, apparently unaware of the serious risk involved, or unconcerned about it.

These drugs appear to work because individual benzodiazepine molecules attach themselves to "receptor sites" in the brain, much as in a child's toy, where round pegs fit comfortably into round holes, and square pegs into square holes. A growing body of scientific evidence indicates that manufactured benzodiazepines mimic similar chemicals that exist naturally in the body. The man-made drugs, research indicates, somehow take the place of the brain's natural tranquilizers and produce results that occur naturally only under special circumstances, such as particular kinds of stress.

The body's benzodiazepinelike chemical has not yet been isolated. When it is discovered, scientists hope it may lead the way to development of tranquilizers with little, if any, potential for abuse and few side effects. (For a more thorough discussion of the way some drugs bind to "receptor sites," see pp. 36–37.)

By directly affecting the brain, benzodiazepines relax the large skeletal muscles, making you either more tranquil or sleepier, depending on the strength of the drug and the amount you take. The drugs are sometimes prescribed to treat fatigue, since fatigue can be caused by overactivity, which may be reduced by a tranquilizer.

Anxiety has been called a normal reaction to the stresses

of life, but some people's day-to-day ability to function is impaired by distressing anxiety. Most physicians would agree that the short-term use of tranquilizers might help them. Depending on each person's particular response to benzodiazepines, and the dosage levels prescribed, the drugs can be useful in treating anxiety for a week to several months. Indeed, some individuals have used them for years with no adverse effects and no significant withdrawal symptoms when the drugs were temporarily discontinued. For most users, however, tolerance builds up and effectiveness starts to wane after about 2 to 4 weeks, and the drugs are better discontinued than increased in large dosage.

Many doctors prefer members of the benzodiazepine family to other, more powerful, sedatives because of their relative safety, fewer side effects, and equal or greater effectiveness. There is little evidence of significant differences between benzodiazepine drugs except for length of action and cost.

Since all benzodiazepines have about the same effect, why is it that Valium, of all the brand names, has attained such a bad reputation for misuse? Some observers of the drug scene say this is because Valium was so well marketed that the name was the one most commonly used both in legitimate circles and during illicit buying and selling. Advertising can indeed work wonders for a drug, just as for a chain of hamburger stands or a model of automobile. A few researchers believe that Valium is possessed of subtle differences that help legitimate users tolerate it slightly better than similar drugs; "on the street," such beliefs were loudly touted by dealers.

That individual benzodiazepines are most commonly prescribed, for example, to treat anxiety but not alcohol withdrawal symptoms—or as a sleeping medication but not for anxiety—is mostly because of advertising and product "positioning" by the manufacturers, rather than real differences between drugs.

Precautions

Do not take these drugs if you know or suspect you are sensitive or allergic to any member of the benzodiazepine group.

Do not take these drugs with alcohol, since the combination can be extremely dangerous.

If you have experienced special sensitivity to alcohol or barbiturates, you may also be unusually sensitive to the effects of benzodiazepines.

Because benzodiazepines may cause drowsiness, you should be careful if you are driving, operating potentially dangerous machinery, or performing some other task that requires concentration and alertness.

These drugs should not be used by anyone experiencing a serious depressive disorder or psychosis.

All benzodiazepines can aggravate narrow angle glaucoma.

Interactions

Benzodiazepines may become extremely dangerous—even deadly—when taken with alcohol; other tranquilizers; narcotics; sleeping pills; barbiturates; monoamine oxidase (MAO) inhibitors; antihistamines; and any other medicines used to relieve depression.

The sedative effects of benzodiazepines may be increased when taken together with cimetidine (Tagamet), which is often prescribed for ulcers.

Smoking may alter the effectiveness of benzodiazepines. Studies show that the percentage of patients feeling drowsy from the drugs is less among heavy smokers.

Common Side Effects

Tiredness and drowsiness at doses suggested for daytime sedation; inability to concentrate; and similar symptoms. Most commonly, users experience mild drowsiness during the first few days of use.

Serious Adverse Effects

Confusion; depression; lethargy; disorientation; headache; inactivity; slurred speech; stupor; dizziness; tremors; constipation; dry mouth; nausea; inability to control urination; changes in sex drive; irregular menstrual cycles; changes in heart rhythm; lowered blood pressure; retention of body fluids; blurred or double vision; itching; rash; hiccups; nervousness; inability to fall asleep; and occasionally liver dysfunction. Frequent use can cause symptoms similar to being drunk.

Occasionally benzodiazepines produce what are termed "paradoxical reactions." While most people are calmed down by these drugs, a small number become extremely excited, fly into rages, and experience hallucinations and increased anxiety.

Dependence and Addiction

If the drugs are taken at several times the prescribed dosage for about a month, physical dependency may develop in anyone; then abruptly stopping the use of these drugs can cause withdrawal symptoms such as seizures.

For most people who take these drugs over long periods of time, there are no significant addiction or withdrawal problems even after months. But among individuals predisposed to addiction, and with a family or personal history of alcoholism, there is a strong tendency to develop severe withdrawal symptoms when stopping the use of even small doses after brief periods of use.

Since there are no significant differences in the effects caused by various benzodiazepines, if you become dependent on one drug you will not alter your dependence by changing to another. If your body becomes tolerant to one benzodiazepine so that ever-increasing doses are needed to attain the same level of sedation, you will be tolerant to all benzodiazepines.

Withdrawal Symptoms

Symptoms of withdrawal, which often occur up to 10 days following the abrupt stop of high doses of benzodiazepines, can include nervousness; anxiety; agitation; insomnia; irritability; diarrhea; muscle aches; convulsions; and loss of memory. Withdrawal symptoms never occur immediately after usage ceases, but may begin in three to five days.

Withdrawal Treatment

Treatment of benzodiazepine withdrawal, which should be medically supervised, usually involves gradually reducing the dosage over a period of several days or weeks. Phenobarbital may be substituted for the benzodiazepine, and then gradually reduced.

Overdose Symptoms and Treatment

Mild overdoses cause drowsiness, mental confusion, and lethargy. More serious overdoses can cause poor muscle coordination; other muscle problems; low blood pressure; deep sleep; and coma.

Overdose treatment includes forcing a conscious victim to vomit and—under medical supervision—maintaining heart activity and breathing.

Anyone suspected of having taken an overdose of benzodiazepines must be taken to a hospital immediately. Always bring the pill bottle so the emergency room staff can quickly identify the medication and begin proper treatment without delay.

Usage in Pregnancy

These drugs should be avoided by women during pregnancy. A child born of a mother using benzodiazepines may face life-threatening withdrawal symptoms during the postnatal period.

If used in the early days and weeks of pregnancy, benzodiazepines may cause defects in the developing fetus. These drugs should also be avoided by women who intend becoming pregnant.

Usage During Breast Feeding

Benzodiazepines are excreted in breast milk. Since infants metabolize these drugs more slowly than adults, and benzodiazepines can therefore quickly build up to toxic levels in infants, they should be strictly avoided by nursing mothers.

Usage by the Elderly

Small initial doses are recommended until tolerance is determined.

Usage by Children

Small initial doses are recommended until tolerance is determined.

BENZODIAZEPINES: ONSET AND DURATION

The chart shows how soon the drugs take effect: the solid lines show peak effect, while the broken lines show the period when most people are affected.

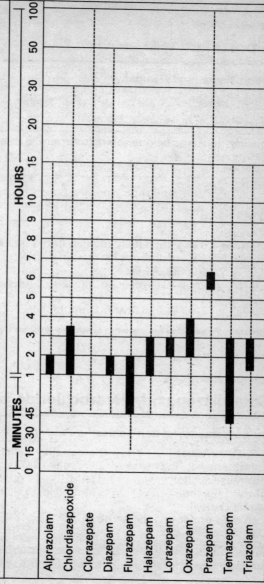

Generic Name

Alprazolam (Schedule IV)

Brand Name (and Company)

Xanax (Upjohn)

Most Commonly Prescribed for

Anxiety; tension; fatigue; agitation; muscle relaxant.

Duration

Short-acting.

Dosage

ADULTS
  0.75 to 1.5 mg. total daily divided into 3 doses gradually increased to a maximum of 4 mg. total daily.
ELDERLY AND CHILDREN
  0.75 mg. total daily divided into 2 to 3 doses gradually increased.
Available sizes: 0.25, 0.5, and 1 mg. tablets.

Important: Precautions and warnings about this drug, pp 185–190

Generic Name

Chlordiazepoxide Hydrochloride (Schedule IV)

Brand Names (and Companies)

A-Poxide (Abbott)
Chlordiazachel (Rachelle)
Libritabs (Roche)
Librium (Roche)
Murcil (Tutag)
Also sold under generic name

Sereen (Foy Labs)
SK-Lygen (SKF)
Tenax (Reid-Provident)
Zetran (Hauck)

Most Commonly Prescribed for

Anxiety; tension; fatigue; agitation; alcohol withdrawal.

Duration

Long-acting.

Dosage

ADULTS

Alcohol withdrawal: 50 to 100 mg. initial dose repeated as needed up to 300 mg. total daily, then reduced.

Mild to moderate anxiety and tension: 15 to 40 mg. total daily divided into 3 to 4 doses.

Severe anxiety and tension: 60 to 100 mg. total daily divided into 3 to 4 doses.

ELDERLY

10 to 20 mg. total daily divided into 2 to 4 doses.

CHILDREN (over 6)

10 to 20 mg. total daily divided into 2 to 4 doses gradually increased to 30 to 40 mg. total daily.

Available sizes: 5, 10, and 25 mg. tablets; 5, 10, and 25 mg. capsules.

Important: Precautions and warnings about this drug, pp 185–190

Generic Name

Clorazepate Dipotassium (Schedule IV)

Brand Name (and Company)

Tranxene (Abbott)

Most Commonly Prescribed for

Anxiety; tension; fatigue; agitation; alcohol withdrawal; seizures.

Duration

Long-acting.

Dosage

ADULTS

Alcohol withdrawal: 30 mg. initially plus up to 60 mg. in divided doses in the next 24 hours. Various dosages next 4 days depending on response, then long-term maintenance dose of 7.5 to 15 mg. total daily.

Anxiety: 30 mg. total daily divided into 3 doses; or single dose at bedtime starting with 15 mg. For long-term usage, 22.5 mg. total daily.

Seizures: 22.5 mg. total daily divided into 3 doses gradually increased to maximum 90 mg. total daily.

CHILDREN (9–12)

Seizures: 15 mg. total daily divided into 2 doses gradually increased to maximum 60 mg. total daily.

Available sizes: 3.75, 7.5, 11.25, 15, and 22.5 mg. tablets; 3.75, 7.5, and 15 mg. capsules.

Important: Precautions and warnings about this drug, pp 185–190

Generic Name

Diazepam (Schedule IV)

Brand Names (and Companies)

Valium (Roche)
Valrelease (Roche)

Street Names

Vals; blues; mother's helper; little violet friend; fives; tens.

Most Commonly Prescribed for

Anxiety; tension; fatigue; agitation; muscle relaxant; alcohol withdrawal; convulsive disorders.

Duration

Long-acting.

Dosage

ADULTS

Alcohol withdrawal: 20 to 40 mg. total first day divided into 3 to 4 doses, then 15 to 20 mg. total daily divided into 3 to 4 doses.

Anxiety, tension, fatigue, agitation, convulsive disorders:
4 to 40 mg. total daily divided into 2 to 4 doses (or 15 to 30
mg. total daily sustained-release capsules).

Muscle relaxant: 6 to 40 mg. total daily divided into 3 to
4 doses (or 15 to 30 mg. total daily sustained-release
capsules).

ELDERLY
2 to 5 mg. total daily divided into 1 to 2 doses gradually
increased as tolerated.

CHILDREN (over 6 months)
3 to 10 mg. total daily divided into 3 to 4 doses.

Available sizes: 2, 5, and 10 mg. tablets; 15 mg. capsules.

Important: Precautions and warnings about this drug, pp 185–190

Generic Name

Flurazepam Hydrochloride (Schedule IV)

Brand Name (and Company)

Dalmane (Roche)

Most Commonly Prescribed for

Sleeping medication.

Duration

Long-acting.

Dosage

ADULTS
15 to 30 mg. at bedtime.
Available sizes: 15 and 30 mg. capsules.

Important: Precautions and warnings about this drug, pp 185–190

Generic Name

Halazepam (Schedule IV)

Brand Name (and Company)

Paxipam (Schering)

Most Commonly Prescribed for

Anxiety; tension; fatigue; agitation; muscle relaxant.

Duration

Long-acting.

Dosage

ADULTS
  60 to 160 mg. total daily divided into 3 to 4 doses.
ELDERLY
  20 to 40 mg. total daily divided into 1 to 2 doses adjusted as needed.
Available sizes: 20 and 40 mg. tablets.

Important: Precautions and warnings about this drug, pp 185–190

Generic Name

Lorazepam (Schedule IV)

Brand Name (and Company)

Ativan (Wyeth)

Most Commonly Prescribed for

Anxiety; tension; fatigue; agitation; sleeping medication.

Duration

Short-acting.

Dosage

ADULTS
  Daytime sedative: 1 to 10 mg. total daily divided into 2 to 3 doses.
  Sleeping medication: 2 to 4 mg. at bedtime.
Available sizes: 0.5, 1, and 2 mg. tablets.

Important: Precautions and warnings about this drug, pp 185–190

Generic Name

Oxazepam (Schedule IV)

Brand Name (and Company)

Serax (Wyeth)

Most Commonly Prescribed for

Anxiety; tension; fatigue; agitation; muscle relaxant; alcohol withdrawal.

Precautions

The 15 mg. tablets contain tartrazine, which can cause allergic reactions in those sensitive to aspirin.

Duration

Short-acting.

Dosage

ADULTS
  Alcohol withdrawal: 45 to 120 mg. total daily divided into 3 to 4 doses.
  Daytime sedative: 30 to 120 mg. total daily divided into 3 to 4 doses.
ELDERLY
  Daytime sedative: 30 to 60 mg. total daily in divided doses.
Available sizes: 15 mg. tablets; 10, 15, and 30 mg. capsules.

Important: Precautions and warnings about this drug, pp 185–190

Generic Name

Prazepam (Schedule IV)

Brand Names (and Companies)

Centrax (Parke-Davis)
Verstran (Warner-Chilcott)

Most Commonly Prescribed for

Anxiety; tension; fatigue; agitation; muscle relaxant.

Duration

Long-acting.

Dosage

ADULTS
    20 to 60 mg. total daily in divided doses.
ELDERLY
    10 to 15 mg. total daily in divided doses.
Available sizes: 10 mg. tablets; 5 and 10 mg. capsules.

Important: Precautions and warnings about this drug, pp 185–190

Generic Name

Temazepam (Schedule IV)

Brand Name (and Company)

Restoril (Sandoz)

Most Commonly Prescribed for

Sleeping medication.

Duration

Short-acting.

Dosage

ADULTS
 15 to 30 mg. at bedtime.
ELDERLY
 15 mg. at bedtime.
Available sizes: 15 and 30 mg. capsules.

Important: Precautions and warnings about this drug, pp 185–190

Generic Name

Triazolam (Schedule IV)

Brand Name (and Company)

Halcion (Upjohn)

Most Commonly Prescribed for

Sleeping medication.

Duration

Short-acting.

Dosage

ADULTS
 0.25 to 0.5 mg. at bedtime.
ELDERLY
 0.125 to 0.25 mg. at bedtime.
Available sizes: 0.25 and 0.5 mg. tablets.

Important: Precautions and warnings about this drug, pp 185–190

CARBAMATES

The tranquilizers known as carbamates include the much-abused Miltown, one of the most popular drugs of the 1950s. Carbamates were the first tranquilizers of their general kind developed by drug researchers, and although their popularity has ebbed somewhat since the introduction of benzodiazepines like Valium and Librium, they still account for more than 200 tons of prescription drug sales each year.

Like benzodiazepines, carbamates affect the brain directly. They relax the large skeletal muscles, and in doing so can make you either more tranquil or sleepier, depending on the drug and how much you use.

Carbamates are most often prescribed as antianxiety drugs, anticonvulsants, or sleeping pills. While they act like short-term barbiturates, carbamates are neither as potent nor as dangerous.

Precautions

Do not take these drugs together with alcohol or other sedatives.

You should not take them if you are allergic to any one of them, or if you suspect you may be allergic to related drugs such as Carisoprodol, Mebutamate, or Carbromal. Because these drugs may cause drowsiness, you should be careful if you are driving, operating potentially dangerous machinery, or performing some other task that requires concentration and alertness.

Those with a family or personal history of drug or alcohol abuse should be carefully supervised when using this drug, since they are at greater risk of developing dependence.

Interactions

In psychotic patients, simultaneous use of tybamate and phenothiazines or other central nervous system depressants has, in a few cases, been associated with grand mal or petit mal seizures. Seizures have been reported with the use of phenothiazines alone, but not with the use of tybamate alone.

Interaction with other tranquilizers, alcoholic beverages, narcotics, barbiturates, other sleeping pills and depressants, or antihistamines, can cause excessive depression, sleepiness, and fatigue.

Common Side Effects

Drowsiness; sleepiness; dizziness; slurred speech; headache; weakness; tingling in the arms and legs; and euphoria.

Serious Adverse Effects

Infrequent: vomiting; diarrhea; abnormal heart rhythms; low blood pressure; itching; rash; effects on various components of the blood; and possibly paradoxical reactions such as excitement or overstimulation. Quite rarely: severe hypersensitivity or allergic reactions producing high fever, chills, closing of the throat (bronchospasm), loss of urinary function, and other severe symptoms. Allergic reactions are usually seen between the first to fourth dose in people having no previous contact with the drug.

Dependence and Addiction

Severe physical and psychological dependence is frequent among people taking carbamates for long periods of time. The drugs can produce chronic intoxication after prolonged use, and if used in greater than recommended doses can lead to adverse effects such as slurred speech, dizziness, and general sleepiness or depression.

Withdrawal Symptoms

Convulsions; tremors; muscle cramps; stomach cramps; vomiting; and sweating. Seizures may also occur in persons with central nervous system damage or preexisting convulsive disorders.

Withdrawal Treatment

Treatment for withdrawal requires extensive medical support care, and must be undertaken in a hospital setting.

Overdose and Treatment

Carbamates have often been used for suicide attempts. Symptoms of suicide attempts or accidental overdose include extreme drowsiness; lethargy; stupor; and coma. Possible shock and respiratory collapse (breathing stops) may also occur.

After a large overdose, the patient will go to sleep very quickly and blood pressure, pulse, and breathing levels will be greatly reduced.

Anyone suspected of having taken an overdose of carbamates must be taken to a hospital immediately. Always bring the pill bottle so the emergency room staff can quickly identify the medication and begin proper treatment, which may include pumping the stomach and other lifesaving measures. Some people have died after taking 30 tablets, while others have survived after taking 100.

An overdose will be much worse if taken together with a large quantity of alcohol or another depressant; in such a situation a much smaller dose of carbamates can produce fatal results.

Usage in Pregnancy

Women should use carbamates with extreme caution if they are in the first trimester of pregnancy, if they suspect they are pregnant, or if they intend becoming pregnant, since these drugs have been associated with birth defects.

Usage During Breast Feeding

Carbamates are found in breast milk, so their use by nursing mothers should be carefully weighed against the possible harm to an infant.

Usage by the Elderly

The elderly are especially sensitive to carbamates and should use them with caution. The same dose taken one time without ill effect may produce excessive depression and be uncomfortable or dangerous the next time.

Usage by Children

Children under 6 should not use carbamates.

Generic Name

Meprobamate (Schedule IV)

Brand Names (and Companies)

Arcoban (Arcum)
Bamate (Century)
Bamo 400 (Misemer)
Coprobate (Coastal)
Equanil (Wyeth)
Evenol 400 (Delta)
F.M. 400 (Amfre-Grant)
Kalmm (Scrip)
Maso-Bamate (Mason)
Mepripam (Lemmon)
Meprocon (CMC)
Meprospan (Wallace)
Also sold under generic name

Meprotabs (Wallace)
Meribam (Merit)
Miltown (Wallace)
Neuramate (Halsey)
Neurate-400 (Trimen)
Pax-400 (Kenyon)
Protran (Vangard)
Robam (O'Neal)
SK-Bamate (SKF)
Saronil (Saron)
Sedabamate (Mallard)
Tranmep (Reid-Provident)

Most Commonly Prescribed for

Anxiety; tension.

Duration

Long-acting.

Dosage

ADULTS
   1200 to 1600 mg. total daily divided into 3 to 4 doses.
CHILDREN (6–12)
   200 to 600 mg. total daily divided into 2 to 3 doses.
Available sizes: 200, 400, and 600 mg. tablets; 200 and 400
mg. capsules.

Important: Precautions and warnings about this drug, pp 200–202

Generic Name

Tybamate (Schedule IV)

Brand Name (and Company)

Tybatran (Robins)

Most Commonly Prescribed for

Anxiety; tension.

Precautions

Contains tartrazine, which can cause allergic reactions in those sensitive to aspirin.

Duration

Short-acting.

Dosage

ADULTS
  750 to 2000 mg. total daily divided into 3 to 4 doses.
CHILDREN (6–12)
  20 to 35 mg. per kg. of weight total daily divided into 3 to 4 doses.
Available sizes: 250 and 350 mg. capsules.

Important: Precautions and warnings about this drug, pp 200–202

HYDROXYZINE

Hydroxyzine, a compound chemically different from benzodiazepines and carbamates, has a similar effect on users. While research has shown to some extent how other tranquilizers work in the body, it is not known how hydroxyzine works.

This drug is used to relieve temporary anxiety such as the stress of dental or other minor surgical procedures. It is also used to relieve the stress of serious but temporary emotional problems, and for the management of anxiety associated with stomach and digestive disorders; skin problems; and behavioral difficulties in children. Hydroxyzine is sometimes used in the treatment of alcoholism.

Precautions

Do not take this drug together with alcohol or other sedatives.

Hydroxyzine should not be used if you know or suspect you are sensitive or allergic to it. Because hydroxyzine may cause drowsiness, you should be careful if you are driving, operating potentially dangerous machinery, or performing some other task that requires concentration or alertness.

Interactions

Hydroxyzine produces excessive drowsiness and sleepiness if used with alcohol, sedatives, tranquilizers, antihistamines, or other depressants.

Common Side Effects

The primary side effect of hydroxyzine is drowsiness, but this usually disappears in a few days or when the dose is reduced. At higher doses, users may experience dry mouth.

Serious Adverse Effects

Tremors and convulsions sometimes occur.

Dependence and Addiction

Unlikely.

Overdose Symptoms and Treatment

The most common manifestation of overdosage is extreme
sleepiness.

If an overdose occurs, vomiting should be induced if it
has not occurred spontaneously, and only if the victim is
conscious. Anyone suspected of having taken an overdose
of hydroxyzine must be taken to a hospital immediately.
Always bring the pill bottle so the emergency room staff
can quickly identify the medicine and begin proper treatment without delay.

Usage in Pregnancy

The use of hydroxyzine is not recommended for pregnant
women, for women who suspect they are pregnant, or
those who intend becoming pregnant.

Usage During Breast Feeding

It is not known whether this drug is excreted in breast milk,
so hydroxyzine should not be used by nursing mothers.

Usage by the Elderly

The lowest effective dosage may be used.

Usage by Children

Permitted in small doses.

Generic Names

Hydroxyzine Hydrochloride
Hydroxyzine Pamoate

Brand Names (and Companies)

Atarax (Roerig)
Hydroxyzine Pamoate (various)
Hy-Pam (Premo)
Vistaril (Pfizer)
Also sold generically as Hydroxyzine Hydrochloride

Most Commonly Prescribed for

Anxiety; tension.

Duration

Short-acting.

Dosage

ADULTS
   75 to 400 mg. total daily divided into 3 to 4 doses.
CHILDREN (6–12)
   15 to 100 mg. total daily divided into 3 to 4 doses.
CHILDREN (under 6)
   15 to 40 mg. total daily divided into 3 to 4 doses.
Available sizes: 10, 25, 50, and 100 mg. tablets; 25, 50, and
100 mg. capsules.

Important: Precautions and warnings about this drug, pp 205–206

3. Narcotic Analgesics

Codeine Phosphate and Codeine Sulfate

Codeine Phosphate with Acetaminophen

Codeine Phosphate with Aspirin and Codeine Sulfate with Aspirin

Codeine Phosphate with Butalbital

Hydrocodone Bitartrate

Hydrocodone Bitartrate Combinations

Hydromorphone Hydrochloride

Levorphanol Tartrate

Meperidine Hydrochloride

Meperidine Hydrochloride Combinations

Methadone Hydrochloride

Morphine Sulfate

Opium Combinations

Oxycodone Hydrochloride Combinations

Propoxyphene Hydrochloride and Propoxyphene Napsylate

For endless hours, under a burning sun, they struggle in the fields to earn the equivalent of a few dollars per day.

With special short-bladed knives, they move from plant to plant making small incisions in the swollen seed pods that stand as tall as their shoulders. Later, they will return to the plants and carefully scrape off the valuable sticky sap that had oozed through each cut.

The plant is *Papaver somniferum*. The opium poppy.

The thick brown substance so faithfully gathered from the seed pods will—through legitimate or illegal channels—eventually be refined into morphine, the basis for many of modern medicine's most powerful pain-killing drugs, and the drug from which heroin is made.

Raw opium has been used for thousands of years. In ancient Greece prescriptions called for the sap of opium seed pods to be dried and compressed, then administered to relieve pain, coughs, and stomachaches. The word we use for these and similar drugs, "narcotics," comes from a Greek word meaning "to make numb."

Morphine was extracted from opium for the first time in 1814, only a few years before the invention of the hypodermic needle. The combination of pure morphine (and, later, other opium derivatives) and the needle ushered in an international age of drug abuse that can be said to have changed the course of the western world.

It is no exaggeration to say that millions, many of them Americans, have died or had their lives critically altered by opium, heroin, or more recent narcotic derivatives.

In the last two decades alone, several hundred thousand narcotic addicts have become criminals to support their habits; babies have been born already addicted because their mothers used heroin; men and women have been gunned down in police shootouts during narcotics busts. The toll in wasted lives and human suffering has been enormous.

Even though only a small percentage of narcotics users become physically dependent on the drugs, virtually anyone who takes them repeatedly will experience some degree of euphoria soon after each dose. This sensation is probably due to the apparent lifting of normal day-to-day worries. Small amounts of narcotics will dampen minor concerns and cause limited euphoria, while larger doses will obliterate more substantial worries and cause greater euphoria. After prolonged usage, however, during which most everyday cares have disappeared, the absence of narcotics can make those worries appear more serious than they seemed before narcotics use began.

There are two sides to narcotics. Their use in relieving severe pain is beyond dispute. Terminally ill cancer patients have been allowed to live their last years, months, or days in dignity without unbearable pain; severely wounded soldiers have survived because of the pain relief provided by narcotics; victims of disastrous accidents have lived because they were not overwhelmed by the pain of their injuries.

In recent decades, naturally occurring opium-based drugs have been largely replaced by a number of derivatives, or synthetics, which contain only a small amount of opium. The derivative drugs, like the originals, not only control pain; they can create a sense of intense euphoria, making them prime candidates for abuse.

Morphine relaxes muscles, causes a decrease in physical activity, and relieves pain and nervousness. When heated together with acetic anhydride, it becomes heroin, a compound developed in 1898 by the same German scientist who later invented aspirin.

Over the past half century laboratories around the world have tried developing the "ideal" narcotic: a drug that relieves severe pain, has no side effects, and is unlikely to be abused or to produce addiction. The search has yet to result in a completely safe pain killer. Some new drugs—like pentazocine hydrochloride (Talwin), a component of so-called "T's & Blues," illicitly used as a heroin substitute—pose particularly serious abuse problems.

Most of the newly discovered drugs have been discarded because they were less effective, or more dangerous, than those already used, but a few stand out as impressive examples of the manufacturing art. Fentanyl, for example, while not available in pill form, has become extremely useful as a preoperative analgesic for open heart surgery, including the world's first artificial heart implant in 1982. The drug provides not only pain relief but a high degree of anesthesia, without many of the serious side effects of other narcotics. But Fentanyl has been widely abused, and after being illegally processed into a compound called alpha methyl fentanyl, is sold illicitly as "China white."

Researchers have discovered that combining certain narcotics like codeine with nonprescription pain relievers like aspirin makes it possible to attain the same pain relief with lower doses of the narcotics. It is not known whether the added ingredients somehow help the narcotics "find" the proper sites within the nervous system where they will have the most pain-relieving impact, or whether the nonprescription ingredients act on pain centers overlooked by the narcotics. Such combination drugs have gained popularity within the medical community since the smaller narcotics dosage extends the time of use before tolerance builds and the drug's effectiveness becomes limited. With large doses of some narcotics tolerance can develop in a matter of days, severely limiting how long they can safely be prescribed.

Opium and opium-based drugs work by directly stimulating receptors in the brain, brain stem, and spinal cord. The molecules of narcotic drugs fit into receptors within the nervous system, like millions of keys into as many locks, to stop pain signals from reaching the brain—or if the electrical impulses do get through, to stop them from being bothersome. A typical comment by hospital patients taking narcotics is "The pain is still there, but it doesn't bother me now." A more thorough discussion of the way narcotics interact with the brain's "receptor sites" can be found in chapter 2.

There are many theories of how pain is experienced, as well as why some people suffer more intensely from a given pain than others. Hundreds of studies have attempted to clarify which pain-killing drug, from aspirin to opium, is most effective in dealing with what kind of pain.

Some researchers are convinced that heroin is the best pain killer ever manufactured, while others believe codeine combined with aspirin or acetaminophen (commonly known by its most popular brand name, Tylenol) is the most effective. Generally, however, it is futile to compare one narcotic pain killer with another, or with a nonprescription drug, since each appears to dampen different kinds of pain, over different time spans, depending on the dosage.

The method of delivering pain killers, according to some studies, may be as critical as the drug or dosage in bringing about relief. British physicians treating terminal cancer patients discovered that smaller doses of pain killers are as effective as large doses if the lesser amounts are provided to patients before each preceding dose wears off. Apparently, because patients never feel extreme pain, they do not develop the subconscious deep fear of pain that will result in their experiencing all pain more intensely.

Most American doctors still prefer to wait until pain returns before allowing their patients to take another pain-killing pill. Out of fear that addiction or dependence will result from too frequent usage, they are considerably more conservative than their British colleagues in prescribing narcotic analgesics. While it is true that frequent use of any narcotic analgesic can result in physical tolerance to the drug (the need for ever-increasing doses to achieve the same analgesic effect), there is little evidence that more than an extremely small percentage of users has trouble stopping use once the medical need is gone. With some narcotics, a mere 48 hours of continual usage can cause withdrawal symptoms if the drug is suddenly stopped, but without a history of addiction—to narcotics, alcohol, or some other drug—there is little chance that an individual will seek more narcotics to ease the pain of withdrawal.

Precautions

Do not take these drugs with alcohol or other sedatives.

Do not take narcotic analgesics if you know you are allergic or sensitive to any of them, or any of their components. Because these drugs are respiratory depressants, use them with extreme caution if you suffer from asthma or other breathing problems. Because narcotics can cause drowsiness and dizziness, you should be careful if you are driving, operating potentially dangerous machinery, or performing other tasks requiring concentration and alertness.

Interactions

Because of their depressant effect and potential effect on breathing, these drugs may become very dangerous when taken together with alcohol; sleeping medicine; tranquilizers; or any other depressant drugs: respiratory depression, low blood pressure, profound sedation, or coma may result.

They should be used with care, and in reduced doses, when taken together with antihistamines; phenothiazines; and tricyclic antidepressants.

Common Side Effects

The side effects of all narcotic drugs are increased by head injury, brain tumor, or other head ailment, and narcotics can hide the symptoms of such illnesses or injury. They should be used with extreme caution in patients with head injuries.

Most frequent side effects include light-headedness; dizziness; sleepiness; nausea; vomiting; loss of appetite (anorexia); and sweating. These effects seem to be more prominent in nonhospitalized users and in those who are not experiencing severe pain. If such effects occur, ask your physician about lowering the dose you are taking. Side effects sometimes disappear if you simply lie down.

Serious Adverse Effects

Respiratory arrest (breathing stops); shock; cardiac arrest; hallucinations; lack of coordination; visual disturbances; dry mouth; loss of appetite; constipation; flushing of the face; rapid heartbeat; palpitations; faintness; urinary difficulties; reduced sex drive; itching; skin rashes; anemia; and yellowing of the skin and whites of the eyes. Narcotic analgesics may make convulsions worse in those who have had them in the past.

Dependence and Addiction

Most people are aware that narcotics have an extremely high potential for abuse and addiction. This varies according to the strength of the individual drug, frequency of use, the circumstances under which it is used, and the susceptibility to addiction of the individual.

The drugs cause relaxation, indifference to pain and stress, lethargy, and euphoria, symptoms making them extremely attractive to addicts. Most people who take these drugs under medical supervision do not develop addiction, but various circumstances—including setting, environment, biological predisposition, attitude, and personality—can combine to produce drug dependence.

There is increasingly well-documented reason to believe that for many people the ritual of "shooting up," or otherwise misusing narcotics, is as important as the potency of the drug in causing addiction. Furthermore, some people who are physically predisposed to do so because of their family or personal history, genetic makeup, or environment become addicts at much lower doses and after using a narcotic much less often. Most people who use narcotics legitimately, even after using large doses over significant periods of time, do not become addicts.

The major signs of addiction include varying degrees of anxiety when the drug is suddenly withdrawn. An addict will go to any length to assure getting another dose, including theft, manipulating doctors with lies and half-truths, and pleading, demanding, and complaining. Most addicts learn, early in their narcotic-controlled lives, the surest and easiest ways to get a continuing supply of drugs.

Withdrawal Symptoms

Sudden withdrawal from a narcotic after lengthy usage usually brings about several extremely severe symptoms, starting with yawning, excessive sweating, and sneezing, and progressing to twitching and kicking movements; tremors; gooseflesh; fever and chills alternating with flushing; anxiety; dilated pupils; overall weakness and aches; loss of appetite (anorexia); nausea; vomiting; diarrhea; cramps; and intestinal spasms.

Withdrawal Treatment

Treatment for narcotic withdrawal, which should be handled only by medical personnel trained to deal with addicts, often includes the use of sedatives to ease anxiety, after which the narcotic is gradually withdrawn over a period of several days. Sometimes a substitute narcotic is given and the substitute is gradually withdrawn. Methadone is often used as a substitute, and after withdrawal is often continued as part of a course of maintenance therapy (see page 227).

Overdose Symptoms and Treatment

It is difficult to define the lethal doses of narcotics, because individuals respond in vastly different ways. Severe overdose is characterized by a decrease in breathing; extreme tiredness; tiny eye pupils; cold and clammy skin; flaccid muscles; and possible coma. Death can result, most often when the drugs were taken by injection.

Overdose treatment, which must be handled in a hospital emergency room, includes reestablishment of an airway (often with breathing controlled by machine); administering drugs that block the action of the narcotic; pumping the stomach if the overdose is from pills; and maintaining a heartbeat.

Anyone suspected of taking an overdose must be rushed to a hospital immediately. Bring the pill bottle so emergency room staff can quickly identify the medication and begin treatment without delay.

Usage in Pregnancy

Narcotic drugs should be avoided as much as possible by pregnant women. Dependence may occur in newborns whose mothers took narcotics during pregnancy. Withdrawal symptoms in newborns include irritability; excessive crying; tremors; hyperreflexia; fever; vomiting; and diarrhea. These symptoms usually appear during the first hours or days of life, and can kill the child if not treated quickly.

Some narcotics are used to relieve pain during childbirth. If they are given to the mother immediately before birth, they will have little effect on the newborn, but if they are administered several hours before delivery, the infant may be seriously depressed at birth and require emergency procedures to stay alive. Narcotics are not recommended when a premature birth is expected, since the newborn may not be able to withstand their depressant effects. The narcotic most commonly used during childbirth is meperidine, in its injectable form rather than as pills.

Usage During Breast Feeding

Narcotics appear in breast milk and can have serious effects on infants, so their use by nursing mothers is not recommended.

Usage by the Elderly

People over 60 are more sensitive to narcotics than other adults; they should take these drugs only under close medical supervision.

Usage by Children

Narcotics should be used by children only when clearly needed, and then only under close medical supervision, since children are more sensitive to these drugs than adults are.

Generic Names

Codeine Phosphate (Schedule II)
Codeine Sulfate (Schedule II)

Street Name

Schoolboy.

Most Commonly Prescribed for

Mild to moderate pain; cough suppressant.

General Information

Codeine phosphate and codeine sulfate, while chemically similar to morphine, produce milder side effects, tending to produce less sleepiness and cause less constipation. Many physicians view these drugs as the best available cough suppressants.

Onset and Duration

Takes effect in 15 to 30 minutes; peaks in 60 to 90 minutes; lasts 2 to 4 hours.

Dosage

ADULTS

Cough suppressant: 10 to 20 mg. every 4 to 6 hours (maximum 120 mg. total daily).

NARCOTIC ANALGESICS: ONSET AND DURATION

The chart shows how soon the drugs take effect; the solid lines show peak effect; the shaded lines, the period when almost everyone is affected; and the broken lines, the period when only some people are affected.

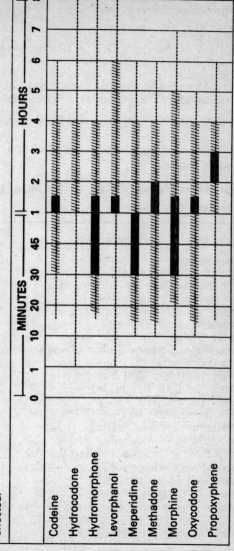

Pain relief: 15 to 60 mg. every 4 hours (maximum 120 mg. total daily).

CHILDREN

Cough suppressant: 2.5 to 10 mg. every 4 to 6 hours (maximum 60 mg. total daily).

Pain relief: 3 mg. per kg. of weight total daily divided into 6 doses (maximum 60 mg. total daily).

Available sizes: 15, 30, and 60 mg. tablets.

Important: Precautions and warnings about this drug, pp 209–216

Generic Name

Codeine Phosphate with Acetaminophen
(Schedule III)

Brand Names (and Companies)

Aceta w/Codeine (Century)
Alorain Tablets (Unitek)
Amaphen w/Codeine (Trimen) (b, c)
Bancap w/Codeine (O'Neal) (b)
Capital w/Codeine (Carnrick)
Codalan (Lannett) (c, s)
Codap (Tutag)
Empracet w/Codeine (Burroughs-Wellcome)
G-2; G-3 (Hauck) (b)
Maxigesic (Merchant) (po)
Omnigesic-C (Delta) (at, br)
Panelex (Delta) (cr)
Papa-Deine (Vangard)
Phenaphen w/Codeine (Robins)
Proval (Reid-Provident)
Rid-A-Pain w/Codeine (Pfeiffer) (a, c, s)
SK-APAP w/Codeine (SKF)
Tega-Code-M (Ortega) (s)
Tylenol w/Codeine (McNeil)
Also sold generically as Acetaminophen w/Codeine

Most Commonly Prescribed for

Mild to moderate pain.

General Information

Combining codeine phosphate with acetaminophen enhances the effect of the codeine without apparently increasing the narcotic's dangers. Some of these pills also contain other ingredients.

Brand names listed above are followed by letters indicating which additional ingredients are present: (a) = aspirin, (at) = acetylcarbromal, (b) = butalbital, (br) = bromisovalum, (c) = caffeine, (cr) = carbromal, (po) = promethazine HCl, (s) = salicylamide.

The aspirin content of some of these drugs may interfere with drugs prescribed to control blood clotting. If you are using such drugs, consult your doctor before taking the medication.

Medications containing butalbital, a barbiturate, can cause barbiturate addiction if taken in sufficiently large quantities over an extended period of time.

Some individuals may be particularly allergic to one of the nonnarcotic ingredients present in many of these drugs; if you know or suspect you are allergic to them, tell your physician before using the medication.

Dosage

ADULTS
1 to 2 tablets or capsules every 4 to 6 hours.

Important: Precautions and warnings about this drug, pp 209–216

Generic Names

Codeine Phosphate with Aspirin
(Schedule III)
Codeine Sulfate with Aspirin (Schedule III)

Brand Names (and Companies)

Anexsia w/Codeine (Beecham) (c)
A.P.C. w/Codeine (various) (c, p)
A.S.A. & Codeine Compound (Lilly) (c, p)
Ascriptin w/Codeine (Rorer) (m)
Buff-A Comp (Mayrand) (b, c)

Bufferin w/Codeine (Bristol) (g, ma)
Empirin w/Codeine (Burroughs-Wellcome)
Fiorinal w/Codeine (Sandoz) (b, c, p)
P-A-C w/Codeine (Upjohn) (c, p)
Rid-A-Pain w/Codeine (Pfeiffer) (c, s)
Tabloid APC w/Codeine (Burroughs-Wellcome) (c, p)

Most Commonly Prescribed for

Mild to moderate pain.

General Information

Combining codeine phosphate or codeine sulfate with aspirin enhances the pain-killing effects of both drugs without apparently increasing the narcotic ingredient's dangers. Since some people are allergic to aspirin, you should be aware of which codeine-based products contain it. Many of these pills also contain one or several other ingredients.

Brand names listed above are followed by letters indicating which additional ingredients are present: (b) = butalbital, (c) = caffeine, (g) = aluminum glycinate, (m) = magnesium aluminum hydroxide, (ma) = magnesium carbonate, (p) = phenacetin, (s) = salicylamide.

Phenacetin, because it can cause kidney damage, will not be included in any of these medications manufactured after August 10, 1983, or sold after August 10, 1984. Drugs containing phenacetin should not be used for more than 10 days because of their effect on the kidneys.

Medications containing butalbital, a barbiturate, can cause barbiturate addiction if taken in sufficiently large quantities over an extended period of time. Some individuals may be particularly allergic to one of the nonnarcotic ingredients present in some of these drugs; if you know or suspect you are allergic to the ingredients, tell your physician before using the medication.

Aspirin may interfere with medications prescribed to control blood clotting. If you are using such medications, consult your doctor before taking pills containing aspirin.

Dosage

ADULTS
    1 to 2 tablets or capsules every 4 to 6 hours.

Important: Precautions and warnings about this drug, pp 209–216

Generic Name

Codeine Phosphate with Butalbital
(Schedule III)

Brand Names (and Companies)

Amaphen w/Codeine (Trimen) (ac, c)
Bancap w/Codeine (O'Neal) (ac)
Fiorinal w/Codeine (Sandoz) (a, c, p)
G-2; G-3 (Hauck) (ac)

Most Commonly Prescribed for

Headache and other pain.

General Information

These drugs combine codeine phosphate with a barbiturate (butalbital) and other ingredients.

Brand names listed above are followed by letters indicating which additional ingredients are present: (a) = aspirin, (ac) = acetaminophen, (c) = caffeine, (p) = phenacetin.

Phenacetin, because it can cause kidney damage, will not be included in any of these medications manufactured after August 10, 1983, or sold after August 10, 1984. Drugs containing phenacetin should not be used for more than 10 days because of their effect on the kidneys.

The barbiturate content of these pills can cause barbiturate addiction if taken in sufficiently large quantities over an extended period of time. Some individuals may be particularly allergic to one of the nonnarcotic ingredients present in some of these drugs; if you know or suspect you are allergic to the ingredients, tell your physician before using the medication.

The aspirin content of some of these pills may interfere with drugs prescribed to control blood clotting. If you are using such drugs, consult your doctor before taking the pills.

Dosage

ADULTS

1 to 2 capsules every 4 to 6 hours (maximum 6 doses daily).

Important: Precautions and warnings about this drug, page 209–216

Generic Name

Hydrocodone Bitartrate (Schedule II)

Brand Name (and Company)

Dicodid (Knoll)

Most Commonly Prescribed for

Moderate to moderately severe pain; cough suppressant.

Onset and Duration

Takes effect in about 1 hour; lasts 4 to 6 hours.

Dosage

ADULTS
Cough suppressant: 5 mg. every 4 to 6 hours.
Pain relief: 5 to 10 mg. every 4 to 6 hours.
Available size: 5 mg. tablets.

Important: Precautions and warnings about this drug, pp. 209–216

Generic Name

Hydrocodone Bitartrate Combinations
(Schedule III)

Brand Names (and Companies)

Anexsia-D (Beecham) (a, c)
Anodynos-DHC (Berlex) (a, ac, c)
Christodyne-DHC (Paddock) (a, ac, c)
Citra Forte (Boyle) (as, c, ch, p, pe, pi, py, s)
Damason-P (Mason) (a, c)
Duradyne DHC (O'Neal) (a, ac, c)
Hycodan (Endo) (h)
Hycomine (Endo) (ac, c, ch, pe)
Norcet (Frye) (ac)
Tussend (Merrell Dow) (ps)
Tussionex (Pennwalt) (ph)
Vicodin (Knoll) (ac)

Most Commonly Prescribed for

Mild to moderate pain; cough suppressant.

General Information

Brand names listed above are followed by letters indicating which additional ingredients are present: (a) = aspirin, (ac) = acetaminophen, (as) = ascorbic acid, (c) = caffeine, (ch) = chlorpheniramine, (h) = homatropine MBr, (p) = phenacetin, (pi) = pheniramine, (pe) = phenylephrine, (ph) = phenyltoxamine, (ps) = pseudoephedrine, (py) = pyrilamine, (s) = salicylamide.

The aspirin content of some of these drugs may interfere with drugs prescribed to control blood clotting. If you are using such drugs, consult your doctor before taking medication containing aspirin.

Phenacetin, because it can cause kidney damage, will not be included in any of these medications manufactured after August 10, 1983, or sold after August 10, 1984. Drugs containing phenacetin should not be used for more than 10 days because of their effect on the kidneys.

Some individuals may be particularly allergic to one of the nonnarcotic ingredients present in many of these drugs; if you know or suspect you are allergic to them, tell your physician before using the medication.

Dosage

ADULTS
  1 to 2 tablets every 4 to 6 hours.

Important: Precautions and warnings about this drug, pp. 209–216

Generic Name

Hydromorphone Hydrochloride (Schedule II)

Brand Name (and Company)

Dilaudid (Knoll)

Street Names

First line; dillies.

Most Commonly Prescribed for

Moderate to severe pain due to surgery, cancer, trauma, colic, heart attack, or burns.

Onset and Duration

Takes effect in about 15 to 30 minutes; peaks in 30 to 90 minutes; lasts 4 to 5 hours.

Dosage

ADULTS
  2 mg. every 4 to 6 hours.
Available sizes: 1, 2, 3, and 4 mg. tablets.

Important: Precautions and warnings about this drug, pp 209–216

Generic Name

Levorphanol Tartrate (Schedule II)

Brand Name (and Company)

Levo-Dromoran (Roche)

Most Commonly Prescribed for

Moderate to severe pain.

Onset and Duration

Takes effect in about 1 hour; peaks in 60 to 90 minutes; lasts 4 to 5 hours.

Dosage

ADULTS
  2 to 3 mg. every 5 to 8 hours.
Available size: 2 mg. tablets.

Important: Precautions and warnings about this drug, pp 209–216

Generic Name

Meperidine Hydrochloride (Schedule II)

Brand Names (and Companies)

Demerol HCl (Winthrop)
Pethadol (Halsey)
Also sold under generic name

Street Name

Cubes.

Most Commonly Prescribed for

Moderate to severe pain; severe migraine headaches; childbirth (usually in injectable form, rather than pills).

General Information

Meperidine is chemically incompatible with barbiturates, and should not be used with them.

Onset and Duration

Takes effect in about 10 to 15 minutes; peaks in 30 to 60 minutes; lasts 2 to 4 hours.

Dosage

ADULTS
  50 to 150 mg. every 3 to 4 hours.
CHILDREN
  1 mg. per kg. of weight every 3 to 4 hours (maximum 100 mg. every 4 hours).
Available sizes: 50 and 100 mg. tablets.

Important: Precautions and warnings about this drug, pp 209–216

Generic Name

Meperidine Hydrochloride Combinations
(Schedule II)

Brand Names (and Companies)

A.P.C. w/Demerol (Winthrop) (a, c, p)
Demerol APAP (Breon) (ac)
Mepergan Fortis (Wyeth) (po)

Most Commonly Prescribed for

Mild to moderate pain.

General Information

Brand names listed above are followed by letters indicating which additional ingredients are present: (a) = aspirin, (ac) = acetaminophen, (c) = caffeine, (p) = phenacetin, (po) = promethazine.

The aspirin content of APC w/Demerol may interfere with drugs prescribed to control blood clotting. If you are using such drugs, consult your doctor before taking this medication.

Phenacetin, because it can cause kidney damage, will not be included in any of these medications manufactured after August 10, 1983, or sold after August 10, 1984. Drugs containing phenacetin should not be used for more than 10 days because of their effect on the kidneys.

Some individuals may be particularly allergic to one of the nonnarcotic ingredients present in these drugs; if you know or suspect you are allergic to them, tell your physician before using the medication.

Dosage

ADULTS
1 to 2 tablets or capsules every 4 to 6 hours.

Important: Precautions and warnings about this drug, pp 209–216

Generic Name

Methadone Hydrochloride (Schedule II)

Brand Names (and Companies)

Dolophine HCl (Lilly)
Methadone HCl Diskets (Lilly)

Street Names

Joice; dolfine; done; dolls; dollies.

Most Commonly Prescribed for

Severe pain; detoxification and maintenance treatment for
heroin addiction.

General Information

Methadone was developed by German scientists during
World War II because they had no access to opium and
desperately needed a pain relief substitute to treat their
wounded. Although chemically unlike morphine or heroin,
it produces many of the same effects, but has a longer
duration of action, up to 24 hours.

Not until the 1960s, after years of experience with methadone in hospitals and clinics, was this drug widely recognized for its usefulness in detoxification and maintenance
treatment programs for heroin addicts.

Addicts are given methadone, even though it is itself
highly addictive, to replace heroin. When dispensed for
this purpose, methadone comes only from government-
approved facilities.

When used for maintenance, methadone, a long-acting
narcotic cross-tolerant with heroin, can eliminate heroin
hunger while causing less drowsiness and fewer other side
effects than heroin, and permitting the user to live a more
normal life. Methadone maintenance often continues for
years. When used for heroin detoxification, government-
approved heroin withdrawal treatment programs using
methadone usually call for gradual withdrawal of the methadone over a period of three weeks or less. If tolerance to
methadone develops, withdrawal symptoms, while usually

less severe than heroin withdrawal symptoms, are usually more prolonged.

Ironically, an extensive drug culture has developed around methadone, the drug selected to control heroin addiction, much like that surrounding heroin. The drug is occasionally stolen from clinics by methadone addicts and sold on the street at high prices. Crimes committed by methadone addicts to pay for the drugs they need have never reached the levels of heroin-related crimes, but are nevertheless widespread. In addition, there is a high incidence of alcohol abuse among methadone maintenance patients.

Onset and Duration

Takes effect in about 10 to 15 minutes; peaks in 1 to 2 hours; lasts 4 to 6 hours, or longer after repeated use due to cumulative effects.

Dosage

ADULTS
   Detoxification: 15 to 40 mg. total daily.
   Maintenance: 20 to 120 mg. total daily.
   Severe pain: 2.5 to 10 mg. every 3 to 4 hours.
Available sizes: 5, 10, and 40 mg. tablets.

Important: Precautions and warnings about this drug, pp 209–216

Generic Name

Morphine Sulfate (Schedule II)

Street Names

Morf; morfina; morpho; morphy; mud; white stuff.

Most Commonly Prescribed for

Severe pain, especially pain associated with heart disease.

Onset and Duration

Takes effect within 20 minutes; peaks in 30 to 90 minutes; lasts 4 to 7 hours.

Dosage

ADULTS
   10 to 30 mg. every 4 hours.
Available sizes: 10, 15, and 30 mg. tablets.

Important: Precautions and warnings about this drug, pp 209–216

Generic Name

Opium Combinations

Brand Names (and Companies)

A.C.D. (Roxane) (at, c, ca, p, s) (Schedule V)
Coldate (Elder) (a, c, ca, p) (Schedule III)
Derfule (O'Neal) (at, p, s) (Schedule III)
Dovamide (Roxane) (at, c, ca, p, s) (Schedule V)
Ricor (Vortech) (ca, po, so, t) (Schedule III)

Most Commonly Prescribed for

Severe pain; diarrhea.

General Information

The use of opium for pain relief has in recent years declined sharply as morphine and codeine have become more popular, but opium is still prescribed frequently to combat diarrhea.

These drugs combine 1.6 to 3.4 mg. of powdered opium with various other ingredients.

Brand names listed above are followed by letters indicating which additional ingredients are present: (a) = aspirin, (at) = atropine sulfate, (c) = caffeine, (ca) = camphor, (p) = phenacetin, (po) = potassium iodide, (s) = salicylamide, (so) = sodium salicylate, (t) = tincture gelsemium.

The aspirin content of some of these drugs may interfere with drugs prescribed to control blood clotting. If you are using such drugs, consult your doctor before taking medication containing aspirin.

Phenacetin, because it can cause kidney damage, will

not be included in any of these medications manufactured after August 10, 1983, or sold after August 10, 1984. Drugs containing phenacetin should not be used for more than 10 days because of their effect on the kidneys.

Some individuals may be particularly allergic to one of the nonnarcotic ingredients present in many of these drugs; if you know or suspect you are allergic to them, tell your physician before using the medication.

Dosage

ADULTS
1 to 2 tablets or capsules every 4 to 6 hours.

Important: Precautions and warnings about this drug, pp 209–216

Generic Name

Oxycodone Hydrochloride Combinations
(Schedule II)

Brand Names (and Companies)

Percocet (Endo) (ac)
Percodan (Endo) (a)
Tylox (McNeil) (ac)

Most Commonly Prescribed for

Mild to moderate pain.

General Information

Brand names listed above are followed by letters indicating which additional ingredients are present: (a) = aspirin, (ac) = acetaminophen.

The aspirin content of Percodan may interfere with drugs prescribed to control blood clotting. If you are using such drugs, consult your doctor before taking Percodan.

These drugs should be taken with milk or after meals.

Onset and Duration

Takes effect in about 10 to 15 minutes; peaks in 60 to 90 minutes; lasts 4 to 5 hours.

Dosage

ADULTS
  1 to 2 capsules every 4 to 6 hours.

Important: Precautions and warnings about this drug, pp. 209–216

Generic Name

Propoxyphene Hydrochloride (Schedule IV)
Propoxyphene Napsylate (Schedule IV)

Brand Names and Companies

Bexophene (Mallard) (a, c, p)
Darvocet-N (Lilly) (ac)
Darvon (Lilly)
Darvon Compound-65 (Lilly) (a, c, p)
Darvon Compound-65 (Lilly) (a, c, p)
Darvon-N (Lilly)
Darvon w/A.S.A. (Lilly) (a)
Dolacet (Hauck) (ac)
Dolene (Lederle)
Dolene AP-65 (Lederle) (ac)
Dolene Compound-65 (Lederle) (a, c, p)
Doraphen (Cenci) (a, c, p)
Elder 65 Compound (Elder) (a, c, p)
Margesic Compound No. 65 (Vortech) (a, c, p)
Pargesic-65 (Parmed)
Pargesic Compound 65 (Parmed) (a, c, p)
Profene 65 (Halsey)
Pro-Pox (Kenyon)
Proxagesic Compound-65 (Tutag) (a, c, p)
Ropoxy (Robinson)
Scrip-Dyne (Scrip)
SK-65 (SKF)
SK-65 APAP (SKF) (ac)
SK-65 Compound (SKF) (a, c, p)
S-Pain-65 (Saron)
Wygesic (Wyeth) (ac)

Street Name

"I've got a yen for that Darvon-N."

Most Commonly Prescribed for

Mild to moderate pain.

General Information

Some of these drugs contain ingredients in addition to propoxyphene hydrochloride or propoxyphene napsylate. Brand names listed above containing other drugs are followed by letters indicating which additional ingredients are present: (a) = aspirin, (ac) = acetaminophen, (c) = caffeine, (p) = phenacetin.

The aspirin content of some of these drugs may interfere with drugs prescribed to control blood clotting. If you are using such drugs, consult your doctor before taking medication containing aspirin.

Phenacetin, because it can cause kidney damage, will not be included in any of these medications manufactured after August 10, 1983, or sold after August 10, 1984. Drugs containing phenacetin should not be used for more than 10 days because of their effect on the kidneys.

Some individuals may be particularly allergic to one of the nonnarcotic ingredients present in many of these drugs; if you know or suspect you are allergic to them, tell your physician before using the medication.

Onset and Duration

Takes effect in about 15 to 60 minutes; peaks in 2 to 3 hours; lasts 4 to 6 hours.

Dosage

ADULTS
  65 mg. every 4 hours (maximum 390 mg. total daily).

Important: Precautions and warnings about this drug, pp 209–216

4. Antipsychotics

Acetophenazine Maleate

Carphenazine Maleate

Chlorpromazine
Hydrochloride

Fluphenazine Hydrochloride

Haloperidol

Mesoridazine Besylate

Perphenazine

Piperacetazine

Prochlorperazine

Promazine Hydrochloride

Thioridazine Hydrochloride

Trifluoperazine
Hydrochloride

Triflupromazine
Hydrochloride

Imagine, if you can, the typical American psychiatric ward of 30 or 40 years ago.

It would remind you of the horrors described in Ken Kesey's *One Flew over the Cuckoo's Nest*. Schizophrenic and other psychotic patients paced aimlessly from bare wall to barred window, and back again. Violent patients were strapped into straitjackets or thrown into padded isolation rooms. Hospital staff members were more like prison guards than medical specialists. And to make things worse, the patient population was steadily increasing, with no end in sight.

Then in the mid-1950s something startling happened. The population of psychiatric patients dropped a little; then the drop suddenly became an avalanche of thousands of patients leaving the hospital wards. And many who remained—the most seriously ill—were increasingly docile. Isolation rooms were used less often. Medical staffers felt relieved as their "guard" duties eased.

Much of the change was due to the development in 1950 of a drug—derived from a chemical, phenothiazine, which had been used by veterinarians for years to kill parasites in animals—called chlorpromazine hydrochloride.

The new drug would be marketed, by Smith Kline & French Laboratories, under the brand name Thorazine.

In 1952 a pair of researchers—impressed by chlorpromazine's apparent usefulness as a presurgery medication—conducted a trial of the chemical among psychotic patients. Their results amazed the international psychiatric community. Most of the experimental patients experienced an unexpectedly high level of relief from the symptoms of their illnesses. News of the results spread rapidly. Patients who just a few months earlier would have been hospitalized could stay home while on the medication. Already hospitalized men and women were beginning to return to their families, since the medications let them function in the community without psychiatric symptoms.

But what about patients who could not be sent home? Had the cloth straitjackets been replaced by chemical restraints? There is still no clear evidence that Thorazine—and similar drugs developed since—cure any of the underlying causes of mental illness. But psychiatric patients in institutions around the world are still given these drugs to alleviate their worst symptoms and, in some cases, to keep them tranquil.

These drugs, which do not lead to dependence and addiction and therefore are not listed in federal drug abuse control schedules, are frequently misprescribed by physicians, leading to misuse. Reports persist of antipsychotics being administered to prison inmates and even to groups of schoolchildren. They are often called "major tranquilizers" because of their overall sedative effects, and to distinguish them from so-called "minor tranquilizers" such as the sedatives (benzodiazepines) and hypnotics (barbiturates), which do not have antipsychotic properties.

Current medical literature persists in recommending antipsychotic dosages that merely subdue patients for the convenience of hospital staffs, without necessarily treating the symptoms of their illness. Haloperidol, a "major tranquilizer" not based on phenothiazine, has become infamous as the drug of choice among Soviet physicians when treating political dissidents who have been diagnosed as psychotic or schizophrenic. In the United States, it is often used in nursing homes.

Antipsychotics are often divided into groups according to their side effects. Some are more likely than others to produce extrapyramidal effects (see "Serious Adverse Effects"); others are more apt to result in anticholinergic effects, i.e., reduction in the amount of stomach acid and slowing of the digestive system. They are also divided according to the levels of sedation they are most likely to produce.

All the phenothiazines have about the same antipsychotic effects and are usually cross-tolerant (if you're extra sensitive to one, you will probably be extra sensitive to all), but some people may exhibit fewer side effects when using one drug than when using another. Antipsychotic effects usually begin from 1 to 4 weeks after therapy starts, depending on the dosage prescribed.

Antipsychotic drugs derived from phenothiazine act on a portion of the brain called the hypothalamus. They affect the parts of the brain controlling metabolism, body temperature, alertness, muscle tone, hormone balance, and vomiting, and sometimes are used to treat problems related to these functions.

These drugs are said to act on the conscious mind much

like a wet cloth thrown on a fire: consciousness is damp-
ened by the drugs, but not snuffed out.

Most of the phenothiazine antipsychotics are legitimately
prescribed for serious psychotic disorders and control of
psychotic agitation or aggressiveness in disturbed children.
They may also be used to relieve nausea; vomiting;
hiccups; restlessness; and apprehension before surgery,
but should only be used in severe cases where less powerful medications have failed.

Precautions

Do not take these drugs with alcohol or other sedatives, if
you suspect you are allergic to them, or if you have any
blood, liver, kidney, or heart disease; very low blood
pressure; or Parkinson's disease. Because these medications are tranquilizers and may reduce alertness, especially
during the first few days of therapy, you should be careful
if you are driving, operating potentially dangerous machinery, or performing some other task that requires concentration and alertness.

These drugs should be used only with extreme caution—
and under strict medical supervision—if you have glaucoma,
epilepsy, ulcers, or any difficulty passing urine.

Avoid exposure to heat and insecticides while taking
these drugs, and avoid sunlight as much as possible, since
antipsychotics increase the skin's sensitivity to light. If you
must be out in the sunlight, use sunscreen lotions on
exposed skin.

Don't use these drugs if you are in a greatly depressed
state or are using any central nervous system depressant,
or have bone marrow depression, subcortical brain damage,
liver damage, jaundice, renal insufficiency, cerebral arteriosclerosis, coronary disease, severe hypotension or hypertension, or mitral valve insufficiency.

Some of these drugs contain tartrazine, which may cause
allergic reactions among those sensitive to aspirin.

Interactions

Phenothiazines should not be taken in combination with
alcohol; barbiturates; sleeping pills; narcotics; other
tranquilizers; or any medication which may produce a de-

pressant effect. Such drugs increase the depressant effects of phenothiazines, as does atropine or drugs related to it.

The use of antidiarrheal mixtures and antacids may reduce the effects of phenothiazines. Antipsychotic drugs may also inhibit the antihypertensive action of guanethidine.

Alcohol should be completely avoided.

Common Side Effects

Drowsiness and dizziness, especially during the first or second week of therapy. If dizziness occurs avoid sudden changes in posture, get up slowly, and use caution when climbing stairs. Urine may become pink or reddish-brown when using these drugs.

Serious Adverse Effects

Phenothiazine antipsychotics can cause jaundice (yellowing of the whites of the eyes or skin), which will usually appear, if at all, within 2 to 4 weeks. The jaundice usually disappears when the drug is discontinued, but there have been cases when it has not. If you notice this effect while taking one of these drugs—or if you develop symptoms such as fever, sore throat, or overall weakness—contact a doctor immediately.

Less frequent serious adverse effects include changes in components of the blood; raised or lowered blood pressure; abnormal heart rates; heart attack; and feeling faint or dizzy.

Phenothiazine antipsychotics can produce what are known as extrapyramidal effects, such as spasms of the neck muscles; rolling back of the eyes; convulsions; difficulty in swallowing; and other symptoms often associated with Parkinson's disease. These effects look very serious but disappear after the drug has been withdrawn; however, a condition known as tardive dyskinesia may persist for several years, especially in the elderly with a history of brain damage. Tardive dyskinesia is generally caused by long-term usage (several months) and is characterized by involuntary movements of the tongue; puffing of the cheeks; mouth puckering; or chewing movements. There is no effective treatment for this ailment. When symptoms of tardive dyskinesia are first noticed, a gradual reduction in dosage sometimes stops the ailment from worsening, but whatever symptoms do occur are likely to continue through life. If you experience either extrapyramidal effects or signs of tardive dyskinesia, contact a doctor immediately.

These drugs may cause hypotension from lowered blood pressure; tiredness; lethargy; restlessness; hyperactivity; confusion at night; bizarre dreams; inability to sleep; depression; and euphoria. Other reactions can include itching; swelling; unusual sensitivity to bright lights; reddening of the skin; and rash.

There have also been cases of breast enlargement; false positive pregnancy tests; changes in menstrual flow; impotence and changes in sex drive in males; stuffy nose; headache; nausea; vomiting; loss of appetite; change in body temperature; loss of facial color; excessive salivation and perspiration; constipation; diarrhea; changes in urine and stool habits; worsening of glaucoma; blurred vision; weakening of eyelid muscles; spasms in bronchial and other muscles; increased appetite; fatigue; excessive thirst; and changes in the coloration of skin, particularly in exposed areas.

Occasionally, sudden death has been reported in patients who have used these drugs. Previous brain damage or seizures may be partly responsible, so high doses of antipsychotics should be avoided by people with a history of seizures. Several individuals who have died showed sudden flare-ups of psychotic behavior shortly beforehand. In some cases, death was apparently due to cardiac arrest; in others, the cause appeared to be asphyxia (choking) due to failure of the cough reflex.

Some of these drugs may block ovulation.

Dependence and Addiction

These drugs do not produce dependence and addiction.

Withdrawal Symptoms

Usually occurring only after high doses are abruptly stopped: upset stomach; nausea and vomiting; dizziness; and tremors. The drugs should not be withdrawn abruptly unless this is required by severe side effects.

Withdrawal Treatment

Treatment of withdrawal symptoms usually includes the use of anti-Parkinson drugs for several weeks after the antipsychotic drug is stopped.

Overdose Symptoms and Treatment

Depression; extreme weakness; tiredness; lowered blood pressure; uncontrolled muscle spasms; agitation; restlessness; convulsions; fever; dry mouth; abnormal heart rhythms; and coma. Anyone suspected of having taken an overdose must be rushed to a hospital immediately. Always bring the pill bottle so the emergency room staff can quickly identify the medication and begin proper treatment without delay.

Treatment for a phenothiazine overdose, which must be carried out in a hospital setting, usually includes maintaining breathing and administering drugs such as anti-Parkinson medications, or diphenhydramine. Vomiting should not be induced, and stimulants, which can cause convulsions, should be avoided.

Usage in Pregnancy

These drugs should not be used during pregnancy, or by women of childbearing potential, except when the potential benefits clearly outweigh any possible hazards, since several side effects have been reported in the newborn.

Usage During Breast Feeding

Safety during breast feeding has not been established, so use is not recommended during lactation except when the potential benefits clearly outweigh any possible hazards.

Usage by the Elderly

The elderly appear to be specially sensitive to these drugs. The most frequent serious side effects among the elderly are restlessness and anxiety, Parkinsonism and tardive dyskinesia. There also appears to be an increased risk of cancer among the elderly using these drugs.

ANTIPSYCHOTICS: SIDE EFFECTS

The chart shows the relative likelihood of side effects from the drugs. For explanations of side effects listed, see text.

	Level of sedative effects	Potential for extrapyramidal effects	Potential for anticholinergic effects
Acetophenazine	moderate	high	low
Carphenazine	moderate	high	low
Chlorpromazine	high	moderate	high
Fluphenazine	low	high	low
Haloperidol	low	high	low
Mesoridazine	high	low	moderate
Perphenazine	low	high	low
Piperacetazine	moderate	moderate	moderate
Prochlorperazine	moderate	high	low
Promazine	moderate	moderate	high
Thioridazine	high	low	high
Trifluoperazine	low	high	low
Triflupromazine	high	moderate	high

Usage by Children

These drugs are seldom recommended for children under 12, and never for children under 2. Children with illnesses such as chicken pox, central nervous system infections, measles, or gastroenteritis, as well as dehydration, seem to be particularly susceptible to adverse reactions.

Generic Name

Acetophenazine Maleate

Brand Name (and Company)

Tindal (Schering)

Most Commonly Prescribed for

Psychotic disorders.

Dosage

ADULTS
   60 to 80 mg. total daily divided into 3 doses (rarely, under close supervision, up to 600 mg. total daily).
ELDERLY
   Lower doses than other adults.
CHILDREN
   Not recommended.
Available size: 20 mg. tablets.

Important: Precautions and warnings about this drug, pp 234–241

Generic Name

Carphenazine Maleate

Brand Name (and Company)

Proketazine (Wyeth)

Most Commonly Prescribed for

Psychotic disorders.

Dosage

ADULTS
   25 to 75 mg. total daily divided into 2 to 3 doses grad-
ually increased to maximum 100 mg. total daily (rarely up
to 400 mg. total daily).
ELDERLY
   Usually smaller doses than other adults.
CHILDREN
   Not recommended.
Available sizes: 12.5, 25, and 50 mg. tablets.

Important: Precautions and warnings about this drug, pp 234–241

Generic Name

Chlorpromazine Hydrochloride

Brand Names (and Companies)

Chloramead (Spencer-Mead)   Promapar (Parke-Davis)
Foypromazine (Foy)   Sonazine (Tutag)
Promachlor (Geneva)   Thorazine (SKF)
Also sold under generic name

Most Commonly Prescribed for

Psychosis; hiccups; nausea and vomiting.

Dosage

ADULTS
   Hiccups: 75 to 200 mg. total daily divided into 3 to 4
doses.
   Nausea and vomiting: 40 to 100 mg. total daily divided
into 3 to 5 doses.
   Psychosis with acute agitation (hospitalized patients): 500
to 2000 mg. total daily in divided doses following initial
injected doses.
   Psychosis with less acute agitation (hospitalized patients):
75 mg. total daily divided into 3 doses gradually increased
to maximum 400 mg. total daily.
   Psychotic agitation, anxiety tension (nonhospitalized

patients): 30 to 75 mg. total daily divided into 2 to 4 doses following initial injected dose gradually increased to maximum 800 mg. total daily.

ELDERLY

Lower doses than other adults.

CHILDREN (over 12)

Nausea and vomiting; psychosis: 0.25 mg. per kg. of weight every 4 to 6 hours.

CHILDREN (12 and under)

Not recommended.

Available sizes: 10, 25, 50, 100, and 200 mg. tablets; 30, 75, 150, 200, and 300 mg. sustained-release capsules.

Important: Precautions and warnings about this drug, pp 234–241

Generic Name

Fluphenazine Hydrochloride

Brand Names (and Companies)

Permitil (Schering)
Prolixin (Squibb)

Most Commonly Prescribed for

Psychotic disorders.

Precautions

Prolixin contains tartrazine, which should be avoided by those sensitive to aspirin.

Dosage

ADULTS

0.50 to 10 mg. total daily divided into 3 to 4 doses (rarely 20 to 100 mg. total daily).

ELDERLY

1 to 2.5 mg. total daily in divided doses.

CHILDREN (over 12)

0.25 to 3.5 mg. total daily divided into 3 to 4 doses.

CHILDREN (12 and under)
   Not recommended.
Available sizes: 0.25, 1, 2.5, 5, and 10 mg. tablets.

Important: Precautions and warnings about this drug, pp 234–241

Generic Name

Haloperidol

Brand Name (and Company)

Haldol (McNeil)

Most Commonly Prescribed for

Psychotic disorders; control of tics; control of Gilles de la Tourette's syndrome (uncontrolled vocal utterances); behavioral problems in children.

General Information

Haloperidol is chemically different from the phenothiazine major tranquilizers, but produces similar results and has the same possible side effects (both common and adverse), interactions with other drugs, and potential dangers.

Precautions

1 mg. and larger sizes contain tartrazine, which should be avoided by those sensitive to aspirin.

Dosage

ADULTS
   Gilles de la Tourette's syndrome: 0.5 mg. total daily gradually increased to 0.05 to 0.075 mg. per kg. of weight total daily in divided doses (rarely higher doses).
   Psychotic disorders: 1 to 6 mg. total daily divided into 2 to 3 doses for moderate symptoms, 6 to 15 mg. total daily for severe symptoms, gradually increased to maximum 100 mg. total daily.
ELDERLY
   Psychotic disorders: 1 to 6 mg. total daily divided into 2

to 3 doses gradually increased to maximum 100 mg. total daily.

CHILDREN (3–12)

Psychotic disorders: 0.5 mg. total daily gradually increased to 0.05 to 1.15 mg. per kg. of weight total daily in divided doses (rarely higher doses).

CHILDREN (under 3)

Not recommended.

Available sizes: 0.5, 1, 2, 5, and 10 mg. tablets.

Important: Precautions and warnings about this drug, pp 234–241

Generic Name

Mesoridazine Besylate

Brand Name (and Company)

Serentil (Boehringer Ingelheim)

Most Commonly Prescribed for

Behavioral problems in children associated with chronic brain syndrome; anxiety; schizophrenia.

Dosage

ADULTS

Anxiety: 30 to 150 mg. total daily divided into 3 doses.

Schizophrenia: 150 to 400 mg. total daily divided into 3 doses.

ELDERLY

Lower doses than other adults.

CHILDREN (over 12)

Behavioral problems: 75 to 300 mg. total daily divided into 3 doses.

CHILDREN (12 and under)

Not recommended.

Available sizes: 10, 25, 50, and 100 mg. tablets.

Important: Precautions and warnings about this drug, pp 234–241

Generic Name

Perphenazine

Brand Name (and Company)

Trilafon (Schering)

Most Commonly Prescribed for

Severe nausea; vomiting; hiccups; psychotic disorders.

Dosage

ADULTS
  16 to 64 mg. total daily divided into 2 to 4 doses.
ELDERLY
  Lower doses than other adults.
CHILDREN (over 12)
  Lowest limits of adult doses.
CHILDREN (12 and under)
  Not recommended.
Available sizes: 2, 4, 8, and 16 mg. tablets.

Important: Precautions and warnings about this drug, pp 234–241

Generic Name

Piperacetazine

Brand Name (and Company)

Quide (Merrell Dow)

Most Commonly Prescribed for

Psychotic disorders.

Precautions

25 mg. tablets contain tartrazine, which should be avoided
by those sensitive to aspirin.

Dosage

ADULTS
  20 to 40 mg. total daily divided into 2 to 4 doses, gradually increased to 160 mg. total daily in divided doses.
CHILDREN
  Not recommended.
Available sizes: 10 and 25 mg. tablets.

Important: Precautions and warnings about this drug, pp 234–241

Generic Name

Prochlorperazine

Brand Names (and Companies)

Compazine (SKF)
Prochlorperazine (Bolar)

Most Commonly Prescribed for

Nausea; vomiting; psychotic disorders.

Dosage

ADULTS
  Nausea, vomiting, psychotic disorders: 15 to 40 mg. total daily divided into 3 to 4 doses.
ELDERLY
  Lower doses than other adults.
CHILDREN (over 2, or weighing 20 pounds or more)
  Psychotic disorders, nausea, and vomiting: (20–29 lbs) 2.5 to 5 mg. total daily; (30–39 lbs) 5 to 7.5 mg. total daily; (40–85 lbs) 7.5 to 10 mg. total daily (rarely up to or slightly more than 25 mg. may be used).
CHILDREN (2 and under or weighing less than 20 pounds)
  Not recommended.
Available sizes: 5, 10, and 25 mg. tablets; 10, 15, 30, and 75 mg. sustained-release capsules.

Important: Precautions and warnings about this drug, pp 234–241

Generic Name

Promazine Hydrochloride

Brand Name (and Company)

Sparine (Wyeth)

Most Commonly Prescribed for

Psychotic disorders.

Dosage

ADULTS
   30 to 1000 mg. total daily divided into 3 to 4 doses.
CHILDREN (12 and over)
   30 to 100 mg. total daily divided into 3 to 4 doses.
CHILDREN (under 12)
   Not recommended.
Available sizes: 10, 25, 50, and 100 mg. tablets.

Important: Precautions and warnings about this drug, pp 234–241

Generic Name

Thioridazine Hydrochloride

Brand Name (and Company)

Mellaril (Sandoz)

Most Commonly Prescribed for

Psychosis; depression; behavior problems in children; multiple symptoms such as agitation, anxiety, depressed mood, tension, sleep disturbances, and fears in elderly.

Dosage

ADULTS
   Depression: 75 mg. total daily divided into 3 doses gradually increased to maximum 200 mg. total daily.
   Psychosis: 150 to 300 mg. total daily divided into 3 doses

gradually increased to maximum 800 mg. total daily divided into 2 to 4 doses.

ELDERLY

Depression, and multiple symptoms of agitation, anxiety, sleep disturbances, etc.: 20 to 75 mg. total daily divided into 2 to 4 doses gradually increased to maximum 200 mg. total daily.

CHILDREN (2 and over)

Behavior problems: 0.50 to 3 mg. per kg. of weight total daily in divided doses.

CHILDREN (under 2)

Not recommended.

Available sizes: 10, 15, 25, 50, 100, 150, and 200 mg. tablets.

Important: Precautions and warnings about this drug, pp 234–241

Generic Name

Trifluoperazine Hydrochloride

Brand Name (and Company)

Stelazine (SKF)

Most Commonly Prescribed for

Psychotic disorders.

Dosage

ADULTS

Psychotic disorders: 2 to 4 mg. total daily divided into 2 doses gradually increased to 40 mg. total daily in divided doses.

CHILDREN (6–12)

Psychotic disorders: 1 to 2 mg. total daily divided into 1 to 2 doses gradually increased to 15 mg. total daily in divided doses.

Available sizes: 1, 2, 5, and 10 mg. tablets.

Important: Precautions and warnings about this drug, pp 234–241

Generic Name

Triflupromazine Hydrochloride

Brand Name (and Company)

Vesprin (Squibb)

Most Commonly Prescribed for

Nausea; vomiting; psychotic disorders.

Precautions

25 and 50 mg. tablets contain tartrazine, which should be avoided by those sensitive to aspirin.

Dosage

ADULTS
  Nausea and vomiting: 20 to 30 mg. total daily.
  Psychotic disorders: 100 to 150 mg. total daily divided into 2 to 3 doses.
ELDERLY
  Psychotic disorders: 20 to 30 mg. total daily gradually increased until effect is optimal.
CHILDREN (over 30 months)
  Nausea and vomiting: 0.2 mg. per kg. of weight total daily divided into 3 doses up to maximum 10 mg. total daily in divided doses.
  Psychotic disorders: 2 mg. per kg. of weight to maximum 150 mg. total daily divided into 3 doses.
CHILDREN (30 months and under)
  Not recommended.
Available sizes: 10, 25, and 50 mg. tablets.

Important: Precautions and warnings about this drug, pp 234–241

5. Tricyclic Antidepressants

Amitriptyline Hydrochloride

Amoxapine

Desipramine Hydrochloride

Doxepin Hydrochloride

Imipramine, Imipramine
   Hydrochloride, and
   Imipramine Pamoate

Maprotiline Hydrochloride

Nortriptyline Hydrochloride

Protriptyline Hydrochloride

Trimipramine Maleate

Tricyclic antidepressants are among the most potent—and potentially dangerous—drugs in use today. Some of them (doxepin and amitriptyline) are considered by experts to be among the dozen or so most abused prescription pills in the nation.

They are most often prescribed for treatment of severe depression, and mixed symptoms of anxiety and depression. They appear to be especially effective in dealing with depression which occurs naturally in some people, due to individual physical makeup. Their use in treating mild anxiety is diminishing, although they are still occasionally prescribed as sedatives.

While the precise way in which they work in the body is unclear—some researchers think they may allow the number of nervous system neurotransmitters to increase (see chapter 2)—tricyclic antidepressants are known to alter mood, improve mental alertness, stimulate appetite, improve sleep, and permit an increase in physical activity.

They produce sedative effects within a few hours after the first tablet or capsule is taken, but their main activity—treating depression—only begins from 4 to 14 days later, depending on which drug is used (see chart on page 256).

To treat depression, these drugs are usually given in gradually increasing doses until a distinct effect is noticed; then the dosage is lowered as much as possible without loss of effectiveness. Patients may be kept on maintenance doses for long periods. The first-day effects, which can include a sense of well-being brought about by the elimination of worries, can make these drugs attractive to people seeking chemical stimulation. Misuse of tricyclic antidepressants, however, stems mainly from physicians' or psychiatrists' inappropriate prescriptions, as when they fail to conduct a thorough examination of a patient and then recommend one of these drugs when some other medication—or none at all—would be more appropriate.

Occasionally these drugs are used to treat nighttime bedwetting in young children, but they generally do not produce long-lasting relief, and such therapy with one of them (doxepin) is of questionable value.

The result of using tricyclic antidepressants without thorough medical supervision can be serious illness or death. Every year, in emergency rooms across the country, these drugs are implicated in hundreds of fatalities, many of them suicides. Some deaths have resulted from combining these drugs with other antidepressants known as MAO inhibitors, or with barbiturates.

Precautions

Do not take tricyclic antidepressants together with alcohol or other sedatives, since they may intensify the effects of the other drugs. Because tricyclic antidepressants may cause drowsiness, you should be careful if you are driving, operating potentially dangerous machinery, or performing some other task that requires concentration and alertness.

Do not take tricyclic antidepressants if you have any reason to suspect you are allergic to them.

Potentially suicidal individuals should not use these drugs. They also should not be used if you are recovering from a heart attack. Tricyclic antidepressants should be taken with extreme caution if you have a history of convulsive disorders; have trouble urinating; have glaucoma; or suffer from thyroid disease. Tricyclic antidepressants increase sensitivity to sunlight; they should be used with caution until the degree of your sensitivity is determined.

Interactions

The interaction of these antidepressants with monoamine oxidase (MAO) inhibitors can cause high fevers, convulsions, even death. Don't take MAO inhibitors until at least 2 weeks after the tricyclic antidepressant has been discontinued.

Alcohol should be strictly avoided while taking these drugs.

Only with extreme caution should tricyclic antidepressants be used together with amphetamines, anticoagulants, sedatives, antihypertensive drugs, and thyroid medications.

Oral contraceptives may lessen the effects of tricyclic antidepressants if used at the same time.

Large doses of vitamin C (ascorbic acid), and smoking, can reduce the effects of these drugs.

The combination of these drugs with large doses of the sedative Placidyl may cause delirium.

Some tricyclic antidepressants contain tartrazine, which may cause allergic reactions in people sensitive to aspirin.

Common Side Effects

Drowsiness; blurred vision; dry mouth; constipation; and difficulty urinating. You should notify your physician if any of these side effects occur.

Serious Adverse Effects

Changes in blood pressure; abnormal heart rates; heart attack; confusion; hallucinations; disorientation; delusions; anxiety; restlessness; excitement; numbness and tingling in the arms and legs; lack of coordination; muscle spasms or tremors; seizures and/or convulsions; skin rash; itching; sensitivity to bright light or sunlight; retention of fluids; fever; allergy; changes in composition of the blood; nausea; vomiting; loss of appetite; stomach upset; diarrhea; enlargement of the breasts in males and females; increased or decreased sex drive; and increased or decreased blood sugar levels.

Less frequent: agitation; inability to sleep; nightmares; feeling of panic; stomach cramps; black coloration of the tongue; yellowing eyes and/or skin; changes in liver function; increased or decreased weight; sweating; flushing; need for frequent urination; drowsiness; dizziness; weakness; headache; and loss of hair.

Dependence and Addiction

Psychological and/or physical dependence is rare.

Withdrawal Symptoms

Abruptly stopping the use of these drugs can lead to nausea, headache, weakness, and an overall sense of not feeling well.

Withdrawal Treatment

There is generally no need for treatment of the mild withdrawal symptoms noted above, other than overall supportive measures, but they should be withdrawn gradually under a doctor's supervision.

Overdose Symptoms and Treatment

Symptoms of overdose include confusion; inability to

concentrate; hallucinations; drowsiness; lowered body temperature; abnormal heart rate; heart failure; large pupils of the eyes; convulsions; severely lowered blood pressure; stupor; agitation; stiffening of body muscles; vomiting; high fever; and coma.

Anyone suspected of having taken an overdose of tricyclic antidepressants must be taken to a hospital immediately. Always bring the pill bottle so the emergency room staff can quickly identify the medication and begin proper treatment without delay.

Because respiratory depression and heart problems can occur suddenly, hospitalization and close observation are necessary even when the overdose is thought to be small. Individuals experiencing heart abnormalities must be monitored continuously for at least 72 hours, well after the heart returns to normal. Even after apparent recovery, relapses may occur.

Usage in Pregnancy

Since tricyclic antidepressants cross the placental barrier, they should be used only when clearly needed, and when the potential benefits clearly outweigh the potential hazards to the fetus.

Usage in Breast Feeding

Not recommended.

Usage by the Elderly

Small initial doses are recommended until tolerance is determined. Those over 60 may become extremely confused during the initial use of these drugs, exhibiting such symptoms as restlessness; agitation; forgetfulness; disorientation; delusions; and hallucinations. The elderly should have regular heart examinations while taking these drugs.

Usage by Children

Children should receive significantly smaller doses than adults. Precise therapeutic doses depend on the child's age, weight, and the effects of initial small doses.

TRICYCLIC ANTIDEPRESSANTS: ONSET AND DURATION

The chart shows how soon the drugs take effect: the solid lines show maximum effect; the shaded lines, the time when most people will be affected; and the broken lines, the time when only some people will be affected.

DAYS

0 1 2 3 4 5 6 7 8 9 10 11 12 13 14 21 30 40 50

Amitriptyline

Amoxapine

Desipramine

Doxepin

Imipramine

Maprotiline

Nortriptyline

Protriptyline

Trimipramine

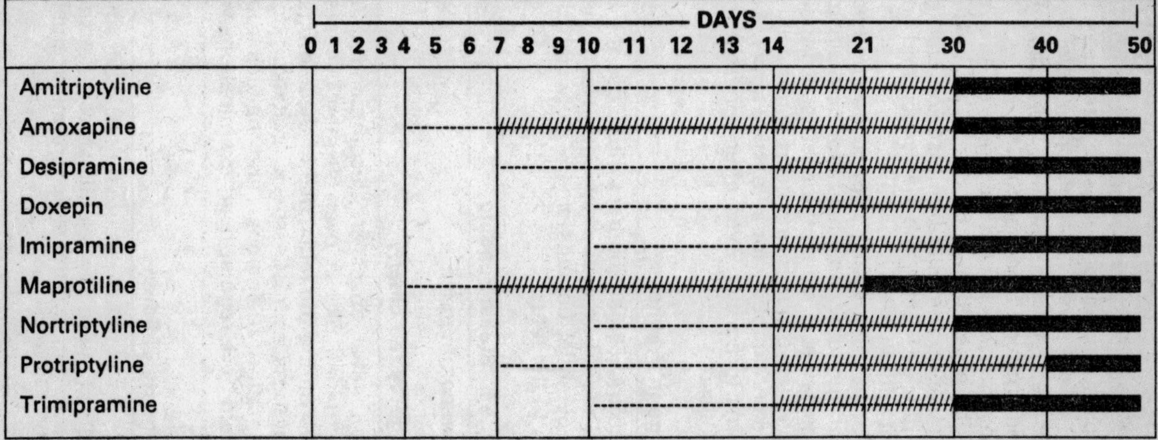

Generic Name

Amitriptyline Hydrochloride

Brand Names (and Companies)

Amitid (Squibb)
Amitril (Parke-Davis)
Elavil (MSD)
Also sold under generic name

Endep (Roche)
SK-Amitriptyline (SKF)

Most Commonly Prescribed for

Depression.

Onset

Response may occur within 10 to 14 days; full effect within 30 days.

Dosage

ADULTS
   75 mg. total daily divided into 3 doses gradually increased up to 150 mg. total daily.
ELDERLY AND ADOLESCENTS
   30 to 40 mg. total daily in divided doses.
CHILDREN (under 12)
   Not recommended.
Available sizes: 10, 25, 50, 75, 100, and 150 mg. tablets.

Important: Precautions and warnings about this drug, pp. 252–255

Generic Name

Amoxapine

Brand Name (and Company)

Asendin (Lederle)

Most Commonly Prescribed for

Depression.

Onset

Response may occur within 4 to 7 days; full effect within 30 days.

Dosage

ADULTS
150 to 300 mg. total daily divided into 3 doses, or a single bedtime dose. Hospitalized patients may receive up to 600 mg. total daily.
ELDERLY
25 to 150 mg. total daily (rarely up to 300 mg.) divided into 3 doses, or a single bedtime dose.
CHILDREN (under 16)
Not recommended.
Available sizes: 50, 100, and 150 mg. tablets.

Important: Precautions and warnings about this drug, pp 252–255

Generic Name

Desipramine Hydrochloride

Brand Names (and Companies)

Norpramin (Merrell Dow)
Pertofrane (USV)

Most Commonly Prescribed for

Depression.

Onset

Response may occur within 7 to 14 days; full effect within 30 days.

Dosage

ADULTS
75 to 200 mg. total daily in divided doses, or a single bedtime dose, gradually increased to 300 mg. total daily.

ELDERLY AND ADOLESCENTS
   25 to 100 mg. total daily in divided doses, or a single bedtime dose, gradually increased to 150 mg. total daily.
CHILDREN (under 12)
   Not recommended.
Available sizes: 25, 50, 75, 100, and 150 mg. tablets; 25 and 50 mg. capsules.

Important: Precautions and warnings about this drug, pp 252–255

Generic Name

Doxepin Hydrochloride

Brand Names (and Companies)

Adapin (Pennwalt)
Sinequan (Roerig)

Most Commonly Prescribed for

Depression with anxiety associated with alcoholism or with major diseases such as cancer which may have a profound psychological effect.

Onset

Response may occur within 10 to 14 days; full effect within 30 days.

Dosage

ADULTS
   Usually starts with 30 to 75 mg. total daily divided into 3 doses, or a single bedtime dose, then gradually increased (rarely up to 300 mg. total daily).
ELDERLY AND ADOLESCENTS
   Lower initial doses than other adults, then gradually increased until effectiveness is determined.
CHILDREN (under 12)
   Not recommended.
Available sizes: 10, 25, 50, 75, 100, and 150 mg. capsules.

Important: Precautions and warnings about this drug, pp 252–255

Generic Names

Imipramine
Imipramine Hydrochloride
Imipramine Pamoate

Brand Names (and Companies)

Antipress (Lemmon)
Imavate (Robins)
Janimine (Abbott)
Presamine (USV)

SK-Pramine (SKF)
Tofranil (Geigy)
Tofranil-PM (Geigy)

Also sold generically as Imipramine Hydrochloride

Most Commonly Prescribed for

Depression.

Onset

Response may occur within 10 to 14 days; full effect within 30 days.

Dosage

ADULTS AND ADOLESCENTS
　75 to 200 mg. total daily in divided doses (rarely 300 mg. total daily) or in a single dose of up to 150 mg. at bedtime.
ELDERLY
　30 to 40 mg. total daily in divided doses.
CHILDREN (over 5)
　Bed-wetting: 25 mg. total daily 1 hour before bedtime increased if necessary to 50 mg. total daily (12 and under) or 75 mg. total daily (over 12), often divided into midafternoon and bedtime doses, then gradually reduced.
Available sizes: 10, 25, and 50 mg. tablets; 75, 100, 125, and 150 mg. capsules.

Important: Precautions and warnings about this drug, pp 252–255

Generic Name

Maprotiline Hydrochloride

Brand Name (and Company)

Ludiomil (Ciba)

Most Commonly Prescribed for

Depression.

Onset

Response may occur within 4 to 7 days; full effect within 21 days.

Dosage

ADULTS
   75 to 225 mg. daily total (rarely up to 300 mg. total daily).
ELDERLY
   50 to 75 mg. total daily in divided doses or as single dose.
CHILDREN (under 18)
   Not recommended.
Available sizes: 25 and 50 mg. tablets.

Important: Precautions and warnings about this drug, pp 252–255

Generic Name

Nortriptyline Hydrochloride

Brand Names (and Companies)

Aventyl HCl (Lilly)
Pamelor (Sandoz)

Most Commonly Prescribed for

Depression.

Onset

Response may occur within 10 to 14 days; full effect within 30 days.

Dosage

ADULTS
  75 to 100 mg. total daily divided into 3 or 4 doses.
ELDERLY AND ADOLESCENTS
  30 to 50 mg. total daily in divided doses.
CHILDREN (under 12)
  Not recommended.
Available sizes: 10, 25, and 75 mg. capsules.

Important: Precautions and warnings about this drug, pp 252–255

Generic Name

Protriptyline Hydrochloride

Brand Name (and Company)

Vivactil (MSD)

Most Commonly Prescribed for

Depression.

Onset

Response may occur within 7 to 14 days; full effect within 40 days.

Dosage

ADULTS
  15 to 40 mg. total daily divided into 3 to 4 doses (rarely up to 60 mg.) or as a single dose.
ELDERLY AND ADOLESCENTS
  15 to 20 mg. total daily divided into 3 doses.
CHILDREN (under 12)
  Not recommended.
Available sizes: 5 and 10 mg. tablets.

Important: Precautions and warnings about this drug, pp 252–255

Generic Name

Trimipramine Maleate

Brand Name (and Company)

Surmontil (Ives)

Most Commonly Prescribed for

Depression.

Onset

Response may occur within 10 to 14 days; full effect within 30 days.

Dosage

ADULTS
  75 to 150 mg. total daily in divided doses (rarely up to 200 mg. total daily) or in a single bedtime dose.
ELDERLY AND ADOLESCENTS
  50 to 100 mg. total daily in divided doses or in a single bedtime dose.
CHILDREN (under 12)
  Not recommended.
Available sizes: 25 and 50 mg. capsules.

Important: Precautions and warnings about this drug, pp 252–255

Sources

"Abuse of Legal Drugs Is Cited." *New York Times* (November 15, 1982): B5.

Alexander, T. "The New Technology of the Mind." *Fortune* (January 24, 1983): 82.

Annas, G.J. *The Rights of Hospital Patients: The Basic ACLU Guide to a Hospital Patient's Rights.* New York: Avon Books, 1975.

Boyd, J.R., ed. *Facts and Comparisons.* St. Louis: J.B. Lippincott Co., 1983.

Cohen, S., ed. *Frequently Prescribed and Abused Drugs: Their Indications, Efficacy, and Rational Prescribing.* New York: Haworth Press, 1982.

Collins, G. "A New Look at Anxiety's Many Faces." *New York Times* (January 24, 1983): A14.

Comprehensive Approach Needed to Help Control Prescription Drug Abuse: Comptroller General's Report to the Congress. GAO/GGD–83–2. Washington, D.C.: GPO, October 29, 1982.

Cornacchia, H.J., D.E. Smith, and D.J. Bentel. *Drugs in the Classroom: A Conceptual Model for School Programs.* St. Louis: C.V. Mosby Co., 1978.

"Department of Health and Human Services, FDA, Weight Control Drug Products for Over-the-Counter Human Use; Establishment of a Monograph." *Federal Register,* Vol. 47, No. 39 (February 26, 1982).

"Depression." *Health Facts* (New York: Center for Medical Consumers and Health Care Information, Inc.) Vol. 2, No. 7, (January/February 1978).

"Diazepam." *PharmChem Newsletter,* Vol. 2, No. 3 (March 1983).

Dorland's Illustrated Medical Dictionary, 25th ed. Philadelphia: W.B. Saunders Co., 1974.

DuQuesne, T., and J. Reeves. *A Handbook of Psychoactive Medicines.* London: Quartet Books, 1982.

Fowler, G. "Addicts Turning To Drug Combinations Cheaper Than Heroin." *New York Times* (December 12, 1982): 56.

Gossel, T.A., and D.W. Stansloski. *Prescription Drugs.* New York: Beekman House, 1981.

Hamilton, H.K., ed. *Professional Guide to Drugs,* 2nd ed. Springhouse, PA: Intermed Communications, Inc., 1982.

"How to Get A Good Night's Sleep—Expert's Advice." *U.S News & World Report* (January 10, 1983): 66.

Hughes, R., and R. Brewin. *The Tranquilizing of America; Pill Popping and the American Way of Life.* New York: Warner Books, 1979.

Inbau, F.E., M.E. Aspen, and G.D. Margolis. *Criminal Law for the Layman: A Citizen's Guide.* Radnor, PA: Chilton Book Co., 1977.

Lader, M., *Introduction to Psychopharmacology.* Kalamazoo, MI: Upjohn Co., 1980.

Long, J.W. *The Essential Guide to Prescription Drugs.* New York: Harper & Row, 1982.

"The Look-Alikes Explosion, Part I." *PharmChem Newsletter*, Vol. 2, No. 3 (May/June, 1982).

Lubasch, A., "Trial Opens for Seven Accused in Sale of Quaalude at 'Clinics.' " *New York Times* (September 25, 1982): 51.

McAuliffe, K. "Brain Tuner." *Omni* (January 1983): 45–48, 115–120.

Mandell, Arnold. "The Sunday Syndrome: A Unique Pattern of Amphetamine Abuse Indigenous to American Professional Football." *PharmChem Newsletter*, Vol. 7, No. 8 (1, 2, 10, 11) (September/October 1978).

Marks, J. *The Benzodiazepines: Use, Overuse, Misuse, Abuse*. Lancaster, England: MTP Press, 1978.

Miller, B.F., and C.B. Keane. *Encyclopedia and Dictionary of Medicine and Nursing*. Philadelphia: W.B. Saunders Co., 1972.

Physicians' Desk Reference, 37th ed. Oradell, NJ: Medical Economics Company, 1983.

The Pill Book. New York: Bantam Books, 1982.

"Psychotropic Drugs: From Valium to Thorazine." *Health Facts* (New York: Center for Medical Consumers and Health Care Information Inc.), Vol. 3, No. 16 (July/August 1979).

Robins, Lee N., Darlene H. Davis, and David N. Nurco. "How Permanent Was Vietnam Drug Addiction?" *The Epidemiology of Drug Abuse*, Supplement, *American Journal of Public Health*, Vol. 64 (December 1974): 38–43.

Sangiacoma, M. "Dr. Zimmerman Headed for Jail." *The Mercury* (Pottstown, PA) (May 15, 1981).

Schnoll, S.H. "Chemotherapy of Pain." *PharmChem Newsletter*, Vol. 2, No. 2 (March/April 1982).

Smith, D.E., and G.R. Gay, eds. *It's So Good, Don't Even Try It Once: Heroin in Perspective*. Englewood Cliffs, NJ: Prentice-Hall, 1972.

Smith, D.E., D.R. Wesson, M.E. Buxton, R.B. Seymour, J.T. Underleidr, J.P. Morgan, A.J. Mandell, G. Jara, eds. "Amphetamines Use, Misuse and Abuse: Proceedings of The National Amphetamine Conference, 1978." Boston: G.K. Hall & Co., 1979.

Sobel, D. "Something Nasty at the Bottom of the Psychiatric Drug Bottle." *New York Times* (June 8, 1980).

Sternbach, L.H., *The Benzodiazepine Story*. Basel, Switzerland: Hoffmann-La Roche Inc., n.d.

Stimmel, B., ed. *Opiate Receptors, Neurotransmitters, & Drug Dependence: Basic Science-Clinical Correlates*. New York: Haworth Press, 1981.

Strauss, S. *The Pharmacist and the Law*. Baltimore: Williams & Wilkins, 1980.

Swain, M. "Valium." *High Times* (March 30, 1982): 30.

Vannini, V., and G. Pogliani, eds. *The Color Atlas of Human Anatomy*. New York: Beekman House, 1980.

Wesson, D.R., and D.E. Smith. *Barbiturates: Their Use, Misuse, and Abuse*. New York: Human Sciences Press, 1977.

———. "Low Dose Benzodiazepine Withdrawal Syndrome: Receptor Site Mediated." *California Society for the Treatment of Alcoholism and Other Drug Dependencies*, Vol. 9, No. 1 (January/February 1982).

Whitaker, B. "Mental Facility, Doctor Sued in Death of Patient." *Kansas City Star* (July 27, 1981).

Wilford, B.B. *Drug Abuse: A Guide for the Primary Care Physician*. Chicago: American Medical Association, 1981.

Index of Generic and Brand Name Drugs

Generic drugs are printed in **boldface** type.

Index of Street Names

ABOUT THE MEDICAL CONSULTANTS

DAVID E. SMITH, M.D., is president and medical director of the Haight-Ashbury Free Medical Clinic, which he founded in 1967. He is also associate clinical professor of toxicology, Department of Pharmacology, University of California Medical School at San Francisco. Long regarded as one of the nation's foremost experts on drugs and drug abuse, Dr. Smith has been a consultant to numerous government agencies and medical and health professionals. Recent programs developed by Dr. Smith include treatment and support for addicted physicians and nurses and cocaine support groups for addicted lawyers, stockbrokers, and other professionals. His first priority remains treating destitute drug abusers in the Haight Ashbury.

Dr. Smith and his colleagues have done seminal research on many facets of drug abuse. The treatment protocols he has developed for stimulants, sedative-hypnotics, PCP, and other drugs are now used throughout the world.

His recent areas of research and training include physicians' prescribing practices, lookalike drugs, benzodiazepines, and amphetamines. He is currently involved in developing national drug-prescribing standards.

Founder and editor of the *Journal of Psychoactive Drugs,* Dr. Smith serves on the editorial boards of several professional journals and has written numerous books and articles, including *PCP: Problems and Prevention; Amphetamine Use, Misuse and Abuse; Drugs in the Classroom; Barbiturates: Their Use, Misuse and Abuse;* and *A Multicultural View of Drug Abuse.* With his colleague Richard Seymour, Dr. Smith writes a monthly consumer information column for *High Times.*

JOHN P. MORGAN, M.D., attended the University of Cincinnati Medical College and trained in internal medicine and clinical pharmacology at the University of Rochester School of Medicine and Johns Hopkins Hospital. He did his residency and internship at SUNY Upstate Medical Center and held a faculty appointment at the University of Rochester School of Medicine before coming to New York City, where he is medical professor and the director of the program in pharmacology at CCNY Sophie Davis School of Bio-Medical Education. He is also associate professor of pharmacology at Mount Sinai School of Medicine, where his specialty is drug misuse and abuse.

RICHARD B. SEYMOUR, M.A., is training director of the Haight-Ashbury Free Medical Clinic and David E. Smith's writing and research associate. As executive administrator, he guided the clinic through the turbulent early 1970s. Mr. Seymour was the first chairman of a statewide California coalition of drug abuse treatment programs and is the current chairperson of the Marin County (California) Drug Abuse Advisory Board. He has been instrumental in the development of physician- and nurse-training courses in drug abuse diagnosis and treatment, prevention, and proper prescribing practices.

A graduate of Sonoma State University, Mr. Seymour has a wide academic background in English and journalism, anthropology and philosophy. Before joining Dr. Smith at the clinic, he worked as a newspaper columnist, cofounded an experimental college, and helped plan the California Open College System. A prolific author, he has written many articles and treatment protocols on drug abuse, in addition to four novels, short stories, and two volumes of poetry. With Dr. Smith, he coauthors a monthly consumer information column on drugs.

Under Mr. Seymour's direction, the Haight-Ashbury Training and Education Project serves health care providers, government agencies, and the general public, as well as a growing number of drug treatment leaders and legislators from abroad. Mr. Seymour is currently preparing a position paper on physicians' prescribing practices and developing physicians' drug-training seminars for use in Europe, South America, and the Far East.